Pediatrics of Common and Uncommon Species

Guest Editor

KRISTINE KUCHINSKI BROOME, DVM, PhD

VETERINARY CLINICS OF NORTH AMERICA: EXOTIC ANIMAL PRACTICE

www.vetexotic.theclinics.com

Consulting Editor
AGNES E. RUPLEY, DVM, Dipl. ABVP–Avian

May 2012 • Volume 15 • Number 2

SAUNDERS an imprint of ELSEVIER, Inc.

W.B. SAUNDERS COMPANY
A Division of Elsevier Inc.

1600 John F. Kennedy Boulevard • Suite 1800 • Philadelphia, Pennsylvania 19103-2899

http://www.vetexotic.theclinics.com

**VETERINARY CLINICS OF NORTH AMERICA: EXOTIC ANIMAL PRACTICE Volume 15, Number 2
May 2012 ISSN 1094-9194, ISBN-13: 978-1-4557-3952-3**

Editor: John Vassallo; j.vassallo@elsevier.com

Veterinary Clinics of North America: Exotic Animal Practice (ISSN 1094-9194) is published in January, May, and September by Elsevier, Inc., 360 Park Avenue South, New York, NY 10010-1710. Subscription prices are $229.00 per year for US individuals, $367.00 per year for US institutions, $117.00 per year for US students and residents, $273.00 per year for Canadian individuals, $433.00 per year for Canadian institutions, $308.00 per year for international individuals, $433.00 per year for international institutions and $150.00 per year for Canadian and foreign students/ residents. To receive student/resident rate, orders must be accompanied by name of affiliated institution, date of term, and the signature of program/residency coordinator on institution letterhead. Orders will be billed at individual rate until proof of status is received. Foreign air speed delivery is included in all *Clinics* subscription prices. All prices are subject to change without notice. **POSTMASTER:** Send address changes to *Veterinary Clinics of North America: Exotic Animal Practice,* Elsevier Health Sciences Division, Subscription Customer Service, 3251 Riverport Lane, Maryland Heights,MO63043. **Customer Service: Telephone: 1-800-654-2452** (U.S. and Canada); **1-314-447-8871** (outside U.S. and Canada). **Fax: 1-314-447-8029. E-mail: journalscustomerservice-usa@elsevier.com** (for print support); **journalsonlinesupport-usa@elsevier.com** (for online support).

Reprints. For copies of 100 or more of articles in this publication, please contact the Commercial Reprints Department, Elsevier Inc., 360 Park Avenue South, New York, New York 10010-1710. Tel.: (212)-633-3813; Fax: (212)-633-1935; E-mail: reprints@elsevier.com.

Veterinary Clinics of North America: Exotic Animal Practice is covered in *MEDLINE/PubMed (Index Medicus).*

Printed and bound by CPI Group (UK) Ltd, Croydon, CR0 4YY
Transferred to Digital Print 2012

Contributors

CONSULTING EDITOR

AGNES E. RUPLEY, DVM
Diplomate, American Board of Veterinary Practitioners–Avian Practice; Director and Chief Veterinarian, All Pets Medical & Laser Surgical Center, College Station, Texas

GUEST EDITOR

KRISTINE KUCHINSKI BROOME, DVM, PhD
Gainesville, Florida

AUTHORS

CHRISTINE ECKERMANN-ROSS, DVM, CVA, CVCH
Avian & Exotic Animal Care, PA, Raleigh, North Carolina

THOMAS C. EMMEL, PhD
Professor of Entomology and Nematology, Professor Emeritus of Zoology, University of Florida; Director, McGuire Center for Lepidoptera and Biodiversity, Florida Museum of Natural History, Gainesville, Florida

RICHARD GLENN HOOD
Retired Licensed Rehabilitator for the US Federal Department of Fish and Wildlife, The Cassowary Conservation Project, Fort Pierce, Florida

JERRY JENNINGS, BS, MBA
Owner, Emerald Forest Bird Garden, Fallbrook, California

JAY D. JOHNSON, DVM
Arizona Exotic Animal Hospital, Mesa, Arizona

ELIZABETH A. KOUTSOS, PhD
Director, Mazuri Exotic Animal Nutrition, PMI Nutrition International, LLC, Gray Summit, Missouri

NADINE LAMBERSKI, DVM
Diplomate, American College of Zoological Medicine; Veterinary Clinical Operations Manager, San Diego Zoo Safari Park, Escondido, California

MARILYN M. MALER, DVM
Instructor of Animal Chiropractic, Options for Animals College of Animal Chiropractic, Wellsville, Kansas; Instructor of Veterinary Acupuncture, Chi Institute of Chinese Medicine, Reddick; Private Practice Veterinarian, SunSpirit Farm and Veterinary Services, Inc., Alachua, Florida

SCOTT G. MARTIN, DVM, MS
Animal Health Clinic, Inc, Jupiter, Florida

ERIN MCKERNEY, DVM
Veterinarian, Peninsula Equine Medical Center, Menlo Park, California

PABLO R. MORALES, DVM
Diplomate, American College of Laboratory Animal Medicine; Associate Director, Department of Veterinary Medicine, The Mannheimer Foundation, Inc, Homestead, Florida

ERIKA NILSON, BS
Pathology and Research Technician, SeaWorld San Diego, San Diego, California

BRUCE A. RIDEOUT, DVM, PhD
Diplomate, American College of Veterinary Pathologists; Director, Wildlife Disease Laboratories, Institute for Conservation Research, San Diego Zoo Global, San Diego, California

APRIL ROMAGNANO, PhD, DVM
Diplomate, American Board of Veterinary Practitioners–Avian Practice; Avian & Exotic Clinic of Palm City, Inc, Palm City; and Animal Health Clinic, Inc, Jupiter, Florida

ANDREA SAUCEDO, MV, RLATG
Research Veterinarian, Occupational Health and Safety Program Manager, Department of Veterinary Medicine, The Mannheimer Foundation Inc, Homestead, Florida

SCOTT SNEDEKER, MD
Diplomate, American Board of Internal Medicine; The Cassowary Conservation Project, Fort Pierce, Florida

JUDY ST. LEGER, DVM
Diplomate, American College of Veterinary Pathologists; Director of Veterinary Pathology and Research, SeaWorld San Diego, San Diego, California

MICHELLE CURTIS VELASCO, DVM
Diplomate, American Board of Veterinary Practitioners–Avian Practice; Fleming Island Pet Clinic, Fleming Island, Florida

MARTIN VINCE, BS
Curator of Birds, Riverbanks Zoo and Garden, Columbia, South Carolina

BARBARA A. WOLFE, DVM, PhD
Diplomate, American College of Zoological Medicine; Vice President of Animal Health, Columbus Zoo and Aquarium and the Wilds, Columbus, Ohio

HUISHENG XIE, DVM, MS, PhD
Clinical Associate Professor, Department of Small Animal Clinical Sciences, University of Florida College of Veterinary Medicine, Gainesville, Florida

Contents

Investigation of all embryo and neonatal mortalities is essential for optimizing productivity in artificial incubation and hand rearing programs. Because artificial incubation is a complex process with many variables, thorough and systematic evaluations are necessary to identify potential problems. Every step of the process from egg lay through incubation and hatching should be evaluated in conjunction with comprehensive data on management of the breeding population. Embryo pathology is one of the most important tools available for identifying disease or management problems in these situations, but it requires extensive background knowledge about avicultural practices and population management.

Psittacine pediatric medicine and surgery can only continue to be practiced by avian veterinarians if psittacine aviculture (the successful captive breeding of parrot species) is active and thriving. Although beautiful, intelligent parrots are popular as beloved pets and reside in zoo and private collections around the world, private psittacine aviculture is in a transition period recovering from difficult economic times. Many of the larger aviculturists have left and the rise of the small aviculturist has significantly changed the industry.

A retrospective analysis of hand-feeding records and growth data from 3 facilities was performed to determine the growth pattern for 8 toucan species raised in captivity. General philosophies of breeding and rearing were similar but approaches to hand-feeding varied. General hand-feeding and chick management records from hatch to fledging were reviewed for 2 of the 3 facilities. Effective hand-feeding formulas were commercially available and minimally modified. Growth curves were developed. Curves approximated typical expected patterns of nestling growth with no loss of weight at fledging. This study provides a basis for hand-feeding protocols and growth curves to assess development.

pathogenic challenges of avian neonates and the associated lesions, avian practitioners can improve their diagnostic and therapeutic success. An area of need for avian research is determining the specific pathogenesis of many conditions affecting avian neonates. By narrowing the specific etiologies, we can improve management and reduce neonatal concerns.

Herpetological medicine and surgery require knowledge and understanding of many different species. Herpetological pediatrics requires even more knowledge and understanding of the differences between adult and neonate, juvenile, and subadult patients. Proper environmental conditions and diet are critical to the health of growing reptiles, and providing the proper conditions and care for hospitalized patients is a vital component of treatment. Challenges often exist due to patient size. Exams, diagnostics, treatments, and surgeries can all be performed successfully on most pediatric patients. Flexibility and some special equipment enable veterinarians to provide high-quality veterinary care to pediatric patients.

Successful breeding of nondomestic ruminants primarily entails meticulous management practices and the prevention of illness through well-planned housing, close observation of dam and calf, and assurance of acquired immunity. Due to the temperament of these species, once a neonate becomes ill, its chance of survival is reduced by the fractious nature of the species and the stress of intensive handling and isolation necessitated by treatment. This article provides strategies for management of the dam and neonate in a nondomestic ruminant breeding program, medical treatment of common conditions, and discussion of the challenges specific to nondomestic species.

In the life cycle of invertebrate animals, the typical life history includes the egg and larval stage, which may be called the pediatric phases, representing development up to the point where the animal reaches adulthood with fully functional reproductive organs and full adult characteristics of morphology, coloration, physiology, and behavior. These typical immature or pediatric stages are found in both terrestrial and aquatic invertebrates. This article reviews the factors that impact the health and survival of juvenile stages of butterflies and moths in particular, and what can be done to extend veterinarian care and advice to clients to invertebrate problems.

> Pediatrics involves a philosophy of comprehensive and continuing
> health care dedicated to the survival and subsequent development of a
> strong, healthy, and well-adjusted infant. Macaque pediatrics plays an
> essential role in any setting whether it be a research setting, display, or
> conservation purposes. This article focuses on macaque infants born
> and raised in captivity. There are multiple parameters that are measured
> and evaluated from birth. Nonhuman primates are usually born during
> the night or early hours of the morning. In an ideal situation, from this
> moment onward, they are cared for by their mothers until weaning.

> The scope of this article will be an introduction to veterinary chiroprac-
> tic and its use in treating pediatric exotic patients. After discussing the
> general principles of human and veterinary chiropractic, the special
> considerations of adjusting exotic pediatric patients will be explored.

> Exotic animals, both pediatric and adult, are amenable to traditional
> Chinese veterinary medicine (TCVM) diagnosis and respond well to the
> TCVM treatment including acupuncture and herbal medicine. With
> more documented clinical experience and experimental studies of the
> TCVM treatment of exotic animals, more diseases in more species will
> be identified to be effectively treated with the TCVM.

VETERINARY CLINICS: EXOTIC ANIMAL PRACTICE

THE CLINICS ARE NOW AVAILABLE ONLINE!

Access your subscription at:
www.theclinics.com

Preface

Pediatrics of Common and Uncommon Exotic Animals

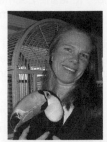

Kristine Kuchinski Broome, DVM, PhD
Guest Editor

Pediatrics has always been one of my favorite aspects of veterinary medicine. As veterinarians, we can have such a profound effect on the future of an individual animal at that point in its life. With exotic species, this can be both challenging and important for the species as a whole. Sometimes a very simple and low-tech solution can take an animal that would be unable to function and survive and allow it to thrive and go onto to a productive life as a pet, display animal, or breeder. I always keep that in mind when hobbling a splay-legged chick or doing a corrective beak trim on a young bird.

As clients become interested in a particular type of exotic, they often view working with that group as a chance to help establish a species in captivity or help maintain the genetics of one that may be endangered in the wild. In that respect, I frequently remind my clients who work with some of the more unusual birds that they really have a responsibility to collect and record as much data as possible about their birds, as much is still being learned. Information is powerful when collected over time. At each facility there will be a unique growth curve for each species that they raise, resulting from their unique combination of genetics, environment, husbandry, and knowledge. Having a record of that lets us discover if an individual baby is falling out of the normal range for that collection and allows earlier intervention in case of a problem. Even in the age of the Internet, too much information about many species remains unrecorded. Recording such data allows them to make a contribution to the knowledge of a species that may lead to more successful reproduction and husbandry in captivity.

The same is true for veterinarians. As we work with some of these exotics, we collect knowledge on many aspects of husbandry and care that should be recorded and made accessible. Some of the most helpful articles can be those in which practitioners share those problems they see on a routine basis and how they specifically treat them. Small tips or tricks can often make a big difference in the outcome of a case. Articles such as these allow us to compile some of what we have learned in a format designed for efficient and widespread dissemination of that

Vet Clin Exot Anim 15 (2012) xi–xii
http://dx.doi.org/10.1016/j.cvex.2012.04.003
1094-9194/12/$ – see front matter © 2012 Elsevier Inc. All rights reserved.

knowledge. I still see many cases that are living with problems that could have been corrected earlier in life or behavioral issues that are essentially created unintentionally by clients. The need is still there to educate owners and other veterinarians on how to treat exotics especially if they are unfamiliar with the species or their husbandry. In mixed species displays we may encounter mammals, birds, reptiles, fish, and butterflies. And, as I am reminded daily, there is always more to learn. Each day we never know when we're going to be surprised with a new client who has something we've never seen.

It was a pleasure to have the opportunity to edit this collection of articles. I would like to thank all the contributors to this issue for their time, enthusiasm, cooperation, and sharing of their knowledge. Thank you also to John Vassallo of Elsevier for all his patience and help with this entire process.

Kristine Kuchinski Broome, DVM, PhD
4508 SE 26th Street
Gainesville, FL 32641, USA

E-mail address:
biffkris@aol.com

Investigating Embryo Deaths and Hatching Failure

Bruce A. Rideout, DVM, PhD, Dipl. ACVP

KEYWORDS

- Embryo pathology • Artificial incubation • Avian disease
- Wildlife

Artificial incubation and hand-rearing allow aviculturists to greatly increase the reproductive potential of breeding populations. When one clutch is pulled for artificial incubation, a second clutch will typically be laid, which can then be parent-reared or also pulled for artificial incubation, thereby doubling or tripling reproductive output. This technique has been used effectively for a number of endangered species recovery programs as well as for a wide variety of domestic and nondomestic birds.[1,2] Because it is important to identify and correct any health or management problems that limit production in these avicultural programs, veterinary involvement makes good financial and conservation sense. Embryo pathology is one of the most important tools available for identifying disease or management problems in these situations, but it requires extensive background knowledge about avicultural practices and population management. This information is not typically available in the veterinary literature, so the essential details are summarized next.

INCUBATION MANAGEMENT

Population-level data on fertility and hatchability for the current and previous seasons are essential for proper interpretation of any mortality. A useful rule of thumb for poultry and other species for which incubation parameters have been optimized is that roughly 80% of the total eggs laid should hatch.[3] Of those that fail to hatch, about 10% should be infertile and 10% embryo mortalities. Mortality or infertility rates above these background levels indicate a problem that warrants investigation. If incubation parameters have not been well worked out for the species, lower hatchability can be expected, but significant deviations from the norm could still indicate an underlying problem that needs to be identified and addressed. These underlying problems typically fall into the categories of incubation management and breeding flock issues.

The author has nothing to disclose.
Wildlife Disease Laboratories, Institute for Conservation Research, San Diego Zoo Global, PO Box 120551, San Diego, CA 92112–0551, USA
E-mail address: brideout@sandiegozoo.org

Vet Clin Exot Anim 15 (2012) 155–162
doi:10.1016/j.cvex.2012.02.005
1094-9194/12/$ – see front matter © 2012 Elsevier Inc. All rights reserved.

Incubation management requires careful control and monitoring of a number of incubation parameters.[4] *Lay-to-set-interval* is the period from lay until incubation starts. In some species incubation begins immediately after lay, while in others incubation does not begin for several days. Large poultry operations often cool eggs for 1 week or longer after lay in order to synchronize hatching, but this is not advisable in other species because extending the lay-to-set-interval can significantly decrease hatchability. Another common practice in the poultry, waterfowl, and game bird industries is cleaning and/or fumigation of eggs prior to setting. Although this can reduce egg bacterial infections in these high-volume operations, such practices are not generally recommended in other species. Cleaning of eggs can remove or damage the cuticle, which is the primary protective barrier against bacterial penetration of the egg, and fumigation can be teratogenic to developing embryos of species with thin-shelled or highly porous eggs (eg, altricial species). Heavily contaminated eggs that are too valuable to be discarded can be gently cleaned with a dry scrubbing pad, being careful to avoid damaging the cuticle. Such eggs should ideally be placed in a separate incubator from other clean eggs.

The amount of *parental incubation* that occurs prior to removal of eggs for artificial incubation is critically important. Eggs with less than 3 to 5 days of parental incubation usually have much lower hatchability and chick survivability.

Proper *setting and turning* of eggs are also very important for hatchability. Eggs from nondomestic species should be set in the incubator in the same position they would be found in the natural nest (poultry have been selected over many generations for successful artificial incubation air cell up). Each egg must be rotated hourly around the long axis. Rotation must be back and forth (continual rotation in one direction winds up the chelaza until they break, allowing embryo to float freely, resulting in mortality). Inadequate or improper turning can increase the incidence of malpositions and embryo mortality. Egg shape is an important consideration when evaluating egg turning problems because rounder eggs are more difficult to keep properly oriented and are therefore more prone to malpositions and embryo mortality. Outlining the air cell with a pencil and placing orientation marks on the egg can help maintain proper positioning during manual turning.

Dry bulb temperature is simply the temperature at which the eggs are incubated. It will vary with the species and is generally determined by the developmental rate of the species. For example, precocial bird species that lay large eggs have a longer incubation period and slower embryonic developmental rate. As a result, they require a lower incubation dry bulb temperature than altricial species that have small eggs with a shorter incubation period and faster developmental rate. An incubation dry bulb temperature that is too high is more detrimental to avian embryos than low incubation temperature, which might only retard development. However, even small temperature deviations can have significant effects. As little as a 0.5° continuous error in incubation dry bulb temperature will result in a significant increase in congenital malformations and embryo mortality.

Relative humidity is based on the incubation dry bulb and wet bulb temperature and is an overall measurement of the humidity in the incubator. Selection of wet bulb parameters for artificial incubation is based on the natural nest microclimate of the species being incubated (eg, humid rainforest species vs dry desert species). Incubation humidity significantly influences egg *weight loss* (water loss), which should be monitored throughout incubation. Eggs are generally weighed every day at the same time and the weight loss is calculated and plotted on a graph. In most species, 12% to 14% weight loss (set to pip) is the target. Abnormal weight loss reduces both hatchability and survivability. Excessive weight loss leads to weak, dehydrated chicks, while inadequate weight loss leads to weak, edematous chicks. Aviculturists will sometimes partially coat the eggshell with nail polish to slow weight loss or sand eggshells to increase weight loss. Glue is also used to seal small cracks in eggs, which could otherwise lead to excessive weight loss, bacterial penetration, or partial loss of egg content. However, coating more than one third of the shell surface can be detrimental and should be avoided.

Incubator *ventilation* is important but can be more difficult to evaluate. Some incubators use still air (without a fan to circulate the air), while others use forced air. Large still air incubators are more likely to develop temperature gradients from top to bottom and require different incubation parameters (dry and wet bulb) than forced air incubators.

There are 45 stages of chicken *embryo development*.[5] With some approximation, this staging system can be applied to altricial species as well. Determining the stage of embryo development at which death occurred (and comparing that to the number of days of incubation) enables evaluation of developmental progress and facilitates formation of a differential diagnosis and diagnostic plan. For example, if the embryo stage is retarded in relation to the days of incubation, it could indicate that the incubation temperature is too low. Based on the fertility and hatchability numbers just given, about 10% of embryos are expected to die during incubation. Typically, there are 2 mortality peaks: one early (prior to stage 25) and one at or near hatching (stages 38–45). In most species, a greater proportion of the mortalities will occur near hatching. Plotting embryo mortalities by stage of development enables one to quickly assess whether an unusual mortality event is occurring.

The chick embryo assumes the proper position to pip (penetrate) the air cell 2 to 3 days before hatch.[6] Lung fluid is resorbed approximately 1 to 2 days before hatch. The air cell is then pipped and breathing begins, resulting in closure of the ductus arteriosus and interatrial foramen and retraction of the yolk sac. At the same time, chorioallantoic membrane blood vessels begin to close down, causing chorioallantoic respiration to decline as pulmonary function increases. The shell is pipped about 16 hours before hatch in the chicken. Hatching proceeds as the embryo extends the pipping hole by rotating within the egg. While the time course of these hatching parameters and the pip-to-hatch-interval vary across species, the data from chickens remain helpful guidelines that can then be adjusted as data become available for the species of interest. Because proper orientation of the embryo in the shell and smooth transition to pulmonary respiration are essential for successful hatching in all species, the hatching period is a critical time for avian embryos.

BREEDING FLOCK MANAGEMENT

Nutritional imbalances, poor body condition, and almost any disease in breeding birds can significantly affect fertility and hatchability of eggs.[7] Clues to nutritional problems include high levels of infertility, poor hatchability, thin egg shells, poor semen quality, egg-binding and other reproductive problems in females, poor plumage, and poor bone quality in chicks. In addition to a thorough diet evaluation, dietary supplements should be investigated. Do not assume that all supplements being used are appropriate or being properly administered. A balanced vitamin and mineral supplement is generally preferred. Nutritional management that includes individual manipulation of vitamin or trace mineral levels can cause problems because the interactions between these micronutrients are complex. Managers may be inclined to individually manipulate nutrient levels if problems with deficiencies have been seen in the past. For example, the author has seen manganese deficiency in nestlings (manifested as slipped gastrocnemius tendons) one season, followed by

100% breeder male infertility in the subsequent breeding season due to manganese toxicosis from oversupplementation. When nutritional problems are suspected, it is important to have access to diet items from the same lots that were being fed during the breeding season, as well as liver samples from affected embryos and archived liver and serum from the breeding flock.

FACILITY MANAGEMENT

When evaluating a facility, pay particular attention to work flow (from clean to dirty) and hygiene practices. Make sure that the disinfectants being used are effective against *Pseudomonas*. Ensure that food preparation for meat-based diets is separate from others and that incubation and hand rearing activities are separated. Water in the reservoirs for humidifying incubators and hatchers should be changed frequently as it quickly becomes contaminated by bacteria, which are then disseminated by aerosolization, contributing to bacterial contamination of eggs and sinus infections in hatchlings. Facility management practices that can increase the risk of infectious disease include a lack of quarantine for new breeders, failure to separate captive and wild eggs, allowing visitors to the facility, poor pest control practices, and allowing workers to have unregulated contact with birds outside the facility (eg, pet birds at home).

INVESTIGATING MORTALITIES

Investigation of individual cases as well as mortality events should proceed in the same systematic way, with all findings interpreted in light of the incubation and population management data. It is very helpful to have the complete history and background data *before* starting the postmortem examination. Record egg weight, length, width, and shell thickness (measured with precision calipers). Assess egg shell shape and quality, smoothness of the shell, degree of surface fecal contamination, and integrity of the cuticle. Open the blunt (air cell) end of the egg with old, dull scissors and evaluate the size of the air cell and slope of the air cell membrane. The air cell increases in size during incubation, typically occupying one fourth to one third of the egg volume by hatching. Examine the membrane itself for evidence of internal pipping or hemorrhage (from vessels lacerated during pipping). Open the air cell with a sterile instrument and obtain a bacterial culture of egg content.

For late stage (near hatching) embryo deaths, carefully evaluate the rotational and postural position of the embryo as it is removed from the shell. The normal hatching position in all species is head under the right wing, with the body oriented so that the beak is pointed toward the lower slope of the air cell (**Figs. 1** and **2**). The 6 possible malpositions are (1) head over the right wing (not usually lethal), (2) head under the left wing (causes moderate to high mortality), (3) rotation away from aircell (moderate to high mortality), (4) leg over the head (high mortality), (5) upside down (high mortality), and (6) head between the legs (high mortality). Keep in mind that positioning is generally only critical in the last 24 to 48 hours before hatch (ie, malpositions are lethal because they prevent pipping and/or hatching; a malpositioned embryo that dies 4 days before hatch most likely died from something other than the malposition alone).

For the external embryo exam, determine the stage of development,[5] evaluate the degree of subcutaneous or generalized edema and look for developmental defects. Examine the yolk sac and allantoic sac membranes carefully for abnormalities. Late embryo deaths occasionally occur when portions of the yolk sac or allantoic sac become wrapped around the head or body during development, preventing the normal movements required for pipping and hatching (**Fig. 3**). Rough handling or improper turning of

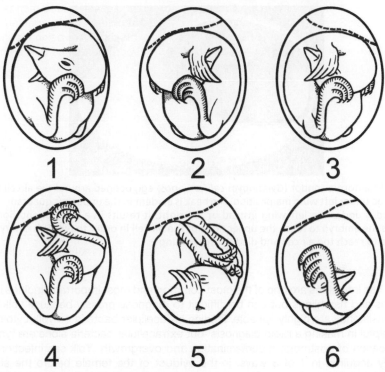

Fig. 1. The six most common types of malpositions in late-stage embryos. (*1*) Head over the right wing (not usually lethal). (*2*) Head under the left wing (causes moderate to high mortality). (*3*) Rotation away from air cell (moderate to high mortality). (*4*) Leg over the head (high mortality). (*5*) Upside down (high mortality). (*6*) Head between the legs (high mortality).

eggs is thought to be an important risk factor. These fetal membrane accidents can also occur in parent-incubated eggs but generally at a lower prevalence.

If the yolk sac is still external, open it with a sterile blade and swab the yolk for bacterial culture and cytology (be careful not to aggressively swab the internal surface of the yolk sac, as hematopoietic cells will contaminate the smears, making it difficult to accurately diagnose an inflammatory process). Limit gross examination of internal organs to evaluating the quantity and nature of the upper gastrointestinal content (which consists of swallowed residual egg content), noting the color, wetness, and degree of inflation of the lungs, and looking for developmental anomalies. Opening very small hollow organs can cause sufficient tissue damage to seriously compromise histopathologic evaluation. Obtain the yolk culture and cytology at this time if the yolk sac is internal.

There are many potential causes of embryo deformities,[3] but incorrect incubation temperature is one of the most important. Evidence in favor of genetic problems would include embryo deformities limited to an individual breeding pair or recurrence of identical deformities in particular pairs but not others. Inbreeding can be an important problem in small populations of endangered species, but be careful about drawing firm conclusions from limited data. Small populations with limited founders will necessarily have pedigrees that could make any problem look hereditary.

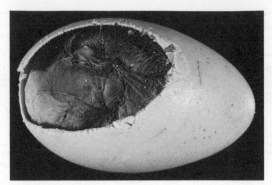

Fig. 2. A California condor (*Gymnogyps californianus*) egg opened around the aircell showing a head under left wing malposition. The beak is evident in the upper left quadrant. When
the head is under the left wing instead of the right, it results in a body orientation that
requires the embryo to reach the upper slope of the air cell in order to pip. This embryo was
not able to reach the air cell and died during pipping.

Yolk sac infections are one of the most common and most important findings in late
embryos and hatchlings but can be difficult to diagnose grossly because yolk color
and consistency are highly variable. Finding intracellular bacteria on yolk cytology is
very helpful in making a rapid diagnosis, but extracellular bacteria alone are typically
an indication of postmortem contamination and overgrowth. Yolk sac infections are
typically acquired in 1 of 3 ways: in the oviduct of the female before the shell is
formed; immediately after lay when air is sucked in through eggshell pores as the egg
cools (which can facilitate bacterial penetration); or during the hatching process when
the umbilicus may be exposed but incompletely sealed. Evaluation of breeding
females, hygiene practices, and pip-to-hatch intervals can help in pinpointing the
source of the problem.

Embryos have little or no inflammatory response until very late in incubation. Even in
late stage embryos, the spectrum of host responses is relatively narrow histologically

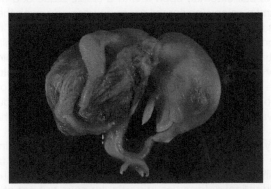

Fig. 3. A stage 44 kea (*Nestor notabilis*) embryo that died during pipping as a result of a fetal
membrane entrapment (the yolk sac is wrapped around the back of the neck). As the yolk sac
began to retract in preparation for hatching, it tightened itself around the back of the neck,
preventing the normal head movements required for pipping. There is prominent edema of
the head and neck accompanying the constriction.

(generally limited to necrosis, heterophilic inflammation, congestion, hemorrhage, and edema). Extramedullary hematopoiesis can be very widespread in tissues, including myocardium. Loose aggregates of mature heterophils in a tissue more often reflect regressing extramedullary hematopoiesis than infection. Chorioallantoic membrane necrosis with mild heterophilic inflammation can be seen in response to normal vascular shut-down during hatch and should not be misinterpreted as evidence of an infection. True bacterial infections will typically have obvious intracellular bacteria and denser masses of heterophils. The most common locations for bacterial infections are the yolk sac and the internal aspect of the umbilicus. Bacteria within the lumen of the proventriculus or gizzard can also be an indicator of in ovo bacterial infections. A small amount of residual lung fluid is normal, but this must be distinguished from aspirated egg content. Congestion, hemorrhage, and edema are relatively common nonspecific lesions.

An infectious process should be ruled out in these cases through cultures and ancillary diagnostics. In the absence of other evidence of infection, these changes only point to the broad categories of incubation and management, genetics (eg, inbreeding), and nutrition. Because the brain of embryos and young chicks is very soft, the entire head should be fixed intact and sectioned for histopathology. This also facilitates evaluation of the nasal cavity and sinuses for evidence of inflammation or aspiration, which are relatively common nonspecific findings in weak hatchlings.

Proper interpretation of gross and histologic findings requires their integration with data on incubation parameters and breeding population management. Some of the common causes of early embryo deaths (stages 1–25) include nutritional problems in breeders, incubation or transport and handling problems, long lay-to-set interval, fluctuating temperatures, power outages or equipment failure, improper turning, poor incubator ventilation, diseases in breeders, in ovo infections, and lethal genetic problems. Keeping in mind that mid-incubation mortality rates should be fairly low, some of the more common causes of mortality in this period (stages 26–37) include egg infections, nutritional problems, and power or equipment failures. The peak in embryo mortality in late incubation (stages 37–45) can be largely attributed to the critical changes occurring just before and during the hatching process. Common problems in this period include malpositions, membrane entrapments, egg infections, and lethal genetic problems. There are many potential causes of death from the time of pipping through 10 days after hatching. These include a lack of sufficient parental incubation, improper turning in the first few weeks of incubation, temperature problems during incubation, humidity problems in hatchers, low oxygen, poor ventilation, hitting a blood vessel during pipping, nutritional problems in the breeding flock, yolk sac infections, umbilical abscesses, and aspiration of egg content.

SUMMARY

Investigation of all embryo and neonatal mortalities is essential for optimizing productivity in artificial incubation and hand rearing programs. Because artificial incubation is a complex process with many variables, thorough and systematic evaluations are necessary to identify potential problems. Every step of the process from egg lay through incubation and hatching should be evaluated in conjunction with comprehensive data on management of the breeding population. The most common sources of significant problems include nutrition and management of the breeding population, insufficient parental incubation prior to artificial incubation, abnormal egg weight loss during incubation, and infections of the yolk sac or umbilicus.

REFERENCES

1. Kuehler C, Good J. Artificial incubation of bird eggs at the Zoological Society of San Diego. Int Zoo Yb 1990;29:118–36.
2. Kuehler C, Loomis M. Artificial incubation of nondomestic bird eggs. In: Kirk RW, Bonagura JD, editors. Current veterinary therapy, XI, small animal practice. Philadelphia: WB Saunders; 1992. p. 1138–41.
3. Romanoff A, Romanoff A. Spontaneous malformations. In: Pathogenesis of the avian embryo: an analysis of causes of malformations and prenatal death. New York: Wiley-Interscience; 1972. p. 17–34.
4. Brown, A. The physical conditions needed for successful hatching. In: The incubation book. Surrey (UK): Spur Publications, Saiga Publishing; 1979. p. 103–44.
5. Hamburger V, Hamilton H. A series of normal stages in the development of the chick embryo. J Morphol 1951;88:49–91.
6. Freeman B, Vince M. Physiology of hatching. In: Development of the avian embryo: a behavioral and physiological study. London: Chapman and Hall; 1974. p. 249–58.
7. Wilson HR. Effects of maternal nutrition on hatchability. Poult Sci 1997;76:134–43.

Psittacine Incubation and Pediatrics

April Romagnano, PhD, DVM, DABVP (Avian Practice)[a,b,*]

KEYWORDS

- Psittacine • Pediatrics • Sexing • Neonatal care
- Diagnostics • Diseases • Psittacine husbandry

As avian veterinarians, we can help by educating our pet bird owners and avicultural clients. We can support our avicultural clients' efforts. We can make an "Aviculturist" binder displaying aviculturists' cards and listing the bird species they breed and sell. We can support and facilitate direct breeder sales. Direct sales result in healthier pet birds as it is safer, for babies especially, to go directly from breeders to their new home.[1]

Education can save many parrots and is very important in today's avicultural climate. The small aviculturist dominates the industry and needs our help. Aviculturists are a group of hard-working individuals who could benefit greatly from well-planned veterinary consults. Some aviculturists keep abreast of husbandry developments but resist preventative medical checkups and nutritional advances, and may even opt to treat many of their sick and injured birds at home. Preventative avicultural medicine can be a tough sell, as it may appear to be a costly process to examine an entire collection, but in the long run, it is more cost effective than triage medicine. The survival rate is much lower with triage or emergency medicine than in a collection with routine preventative medicine. Although small aviculturists can be seasoned and knowledgeable, as mentioned, they are more commonly isolated, uninformed, and eager to learn. Avian veterinarians can make a difference by focusing on avicultural education and pediatrics. This is important because aviculture is the only future for many parrot species. Further, aviculturists' predominantly have their birds' best interests at heart and most are very receptive to new ideas. This is especially true if we, as avian veterinarians, take the time, on a regular basis, to educate them, answer their questions, and address their concerns.

Like psittacine pediatric medicine and surgery, a significant part of avicultural medicine is HUSBANDRY, and the most important husbandry issue is nutrition.[1] Nutrition is important at all levels of psittacine development. Hence, the avian

The author has nothing to disclose.
[a] Avian & Exotic Clinic of Palm City, Inc, 4181 SW High Meadow Avenue, Palm City, FL 34990, USA
[b] Animal Health Clinic, Inc, 5500 Military Trail, Suite #40, Jupiter, FL 33458, USA
* Avian & Exotic Clinic of Palm City, Inc, 4181 SW High Meadow Avenue, Palm City, FL 34990.
E-mail address: draprilr@aol.com

Vet Clin Exot Anim 15 (2012) 163–182
http://dx.doi.org/10.1016/j.cvex.2012.04.002
1094-9194/12/$ – see front matter © 2012 Elsevier Inc. All rights reserved.

veterinarian must become knowledgeable of neonatal and juvenile handfeeding formulas and techniques, weaning feeds, adult and breeder bird pellets, as well as specific nutritional requirements of parrots of all ages.

Avian veterinarians must be readily available, in the author's opinion, on a 24-hour-a-day basis. They must also take the time to educate their avicultural and baby bird clients, both individually and in groups. Education can take place within the clinic, on site at breeding facilities, or at bird clubs and national meetings. The important thing is to educate, consult, listen, and help these people and consequently help their birds.

The first requirement for successful captive breeding is a true pair.[2] Gender determination is paramount for successful psittacine aviculture. Sexing is necessary because psittacines are predominantly monomorphic. This has resulted in many same-sex pairs, thought to be true pairs, inadvertently set up for years.[2] This is especially true when a female pair is producing eggs. Accurate sex determination is also important because sexing is a veterinary service and the avian veterinarian is making a diagnosis. Various options for sexing are available; hence the avian veterinarian can choose the method most suitable to the patient and the client. Additionally, sexing of baby birds can help breeders who wish to sell their birds as a particular gender at an early age.

SEXING
Visual Sexing

A few psittacine species are sexually dimorphic and can be definitively sexed by visual examination. Some examples follow:

- Eclectus parrot: Males are green and females are vibrant red and purple.
- White-fronted Amazon parrot: Males have red versus green feathers on the upper wing coverts, the edge of the carpus, and the alula.
- Pileated parrot: Males have red feathers on head, and females has green.
- Red-tailed black cockatoos: Females have spots on head, body, and wing feathers, and the tail is barred with yellow-orange feathers. Males lack spots and the tail has red bars.
- White-tailed black cockatoos: Females have white ear coverts and light horn-colored beak. Males have gray ear coverts and dark gray beaks.
- Gang-gang cockatoos: Males have red head and crest feathers, and females are totally gray, barred with grayish white.
- Pesquet's parrot: Males have red feathers behind the eye, which are absent in females.
- Australian king parrot: The males have scarlet red feathers on the head, neck, and under parts. Females have green feathers on the head and chest and red feathers on the lower abdomen. The beak is red-orange and black tipped in the male and black in the female.

Vent Sexing

Vent sexing is an accurate sexing method for one psittacine species, the Vasa parrot, where a penis-like appendage is found in male birds.

Surgical Sexing

First performed in the 1970s, surgical sexing is by far the best and most direct method of gender determination in monomorphic psittacine birds of almost any age. The main disadvantage of surgical sexing is the inherent, though minimal, surgical and anesthetic risk. The advantages of surgical sexing are many, including a complete visual assessment of the internal organs on the left side of the bird's body as well as assessing the birds for internal disease.

Cytogenetic Sexing

First performed in the 1980s, cytogenetic sexing is a nonsurgical alternative for sexing birds. A freshly plucked contour blood feather is the preferred source of chromosomal DNA in psittacine birds. The plucked feather is immediately placed in media for overnight mailing to a cytogenetic laboratory. Chromosomal analysis is performed on cells cultured from the submitted feather.[3]

Advantages of cytogenetics include karyotype evaluation and identification of chromosomal defects. Cytogenetic defects identified in psittacines include chromosomal inversions, chromosome translocations, triploidy, and ZZ ZW chimerism. These defects significantly reduce fertility. Disadvantages of feather sexing include a 2-week turnaround time and the possibility of culture failure.[3]

DNA Sexing

First commercially available in the 1990s, the newest means of nonsurgical sex determination in avian medicine is DNA sexing. This technique involves acquiring and submitting a small amount of whole blood or a few blood feathers to a laboratory. The DNA is run on an electrophoretic gel (Southern blot), and the resulting bands are probed and compared with male and female controls. The main disadvantages of DNA sexing is the turnaround time, the lack of species-specific probes in some cases, and the possibility of error due to sample mixup or sample contamination with DNA from a bird of the opposite sex.

INCUBATION AND HATCHING

Successful incubation and hatching require intensive husbandry. Similarly, altricial psittacine chicks require intensive care from day 1. Neonates hatch with eyes closed and little to no down and are unable to thermoregulate, and they need to be hand-fed.[4–7] Thus, in addition to preventative and triage medicine, the avian veterinarian can help the aviculturist by evaluating the following processes: incubation, hatching, handfeeding, neonatal development, and weaning.

Natural incubation by captive psittacines is affected by many factors, including demonstration of normal breeding behaviors by both parents, health, diet, species, origin (wild caught or hand raised), experience, environment, egg integrity, and nest box design.[6,8] Perhaps the most important of these is the demonstration of normal breeding behaviors. The female should act broody and prepare for and care for her nest of eggs. The nest should be prepared with the help of her mate and be kept clean and well protected.[6] The male should take on the role of provider and feed the female consistently throughout the pre–egg-laying and post–egg-laying periods. One or both of the parents may feed the offspring. Males are known to lose weight during this time as they are passing the nutrition on to their mate and offspring.[6]

Nest box parameters such as cleanliness, shape, depth, width, height, and degree of openness and the amount of lighting are important for breeding success.[8] Broken or cracked eggs are susceptible to bacterial or fungal infections, and should be repaired with nail polish and incubated artificially.[6]

Hatchability of artificially incubated eggs pulled at day 1 is lower than that for eggs naturally incubated for the first 7 to 14 days.[6] Further, large psittacine eggs seem to be more tolerant of incubation from day 1 than are the eggs of smaller psittacine species. Incubation of eggs from day 1 is tedious and time consuming but frequently increases overall production from the pair. This increase occurs despite increased individual egg loss because pulling the eggs at day 1 encourages the hen to lay again, thus increasing the number of eggs laid per clutch, as well as the number of clutches laid per year. Birds should not be encouraged to clutch more than 2 or 3 times a year.

Successful artificial incubation is dependent on several parameters including temperature, humidity, airflow in the incubator or hatcher, vibration, and egg rotation. Egg rotation is very important in artificial incubation. It is required to prevent embryo adhesion to the shell membranes. Parents will turn their eggs every 35 minutes.[6] Inadequate turning in artificial incubation results in early-dead-in-shell, malpositioned, or late-dead-in-shell embryos. Good-quality commercial incubators turn eggs at different rates on various types of timed mechanical rollers, with 10 turns per day being the average.[6] A minimum of 5 turns per day is required in machines where automatic turning is not an option.[6] A popular and reliable artificial incubator is the Grumbach (Grumbach, Assalar, Germany). Artificial incubators and hatchers should be cultured for bacteria and fungi several times a year, as well as a DNA probe tested for polyoma and psittacine beak and feather virus. Units should also be cleaned and gas sterilized yearly at a minimum, whenever empty or ideally between sets of eggs.

Incubation temperature and humidity vary for different psittacine species but range from 98.9° to 99.3°F (37.3°C) and 30% to 45%, respectively. Digital hygrometers work best to monitor humidity. Incubation room temperature is ideally maintained at 73° to 75°F (22.5°C) with a humidity of 43% to 48%. Most psittacine embryos are best hatched at 99.5°F (37.5°C) with a hygrometer reading of 65% to 75%.[6]

Artificially incubated eggs are candled to monitor development and should be moved to the bottom of the incubator and no longer turned once draw down has been noted, as this is when internal pipping begins. A simple small flashlight can be used for candling. Some aviculturists will candle daily, but the majority candle weekly or biweekly as psittacine eggs are less tolerant of handling than are poultry eggs. However, candling, a necessary form of handling, is important in determining embryo fertility and viability. The critical periods of development for psittacines are the first few days of incubation and the time from internal pip until hatching.[6] During these times, the embryo is most susceptible to adverse handling and/or improper incubation parameters. Incubation times vary for different psittacine species and range from approximately 18 days in budgerigars to approximately 30 days in palm cockatoos.

The first sign of fertility are blood vessels radiating uniformly from the embryo in a branching pattern around day 4 or 5 in some species, but they can be seen as early as 3 days. Eggs with clear yolks showing no signs of blood vessels or development by day 7 are infertile, or early dead in shell, and should be removed from the incubator (or nest). A healthy developing psittacine egg should lose between 11% and 16% (average 13%) of its water weight by diffusion during incubation (day 1 to external pip). The air cell should form at the larger rounded end of the egg during this period of weight loss. If the humidity is too high, however, the air cell will be small, and if it is too low, then the air cell will be larger. Washing of eggs, typically done in the poultry industry, is thought to be risky for psittacine eggs and is not recommended.[6]

The normal psittacine embryo assumes the hatching position with its head below the air cell just before hatching. Psittacine embryos have shorter and thicker necks than chicken embryos and do not normally tuck their heads under their right wing.[6] Instead, they barely tuck their head and typically lay it close to the right wing tip. Hatching occurs in stages (draw down, internal pip, external pip, emergence from the egg) and is the time of highest mortality in embryonic development. Approximately 24 to 48 hours prior to internal pip, the air cell expands and extends down, or draws down, one side of the egg, occupying 20% to 30 % of its volume. An increase in the level of carbon dioxide (CO_2) then occurs because the gaseous exchange needs of the embryo are no longer met by the allantoic circulation. This build-up of CO_2 causes the hatching muscle in the neck to twitch. This twitch causes the egg tooth, which is located rostrally on the tip of the maxilla, to penetrate the chorioallantoic membrane (ie, internal pip). At this point, the embryo becomes a chick, as it begins to breathe air within the air cell. As the lungs begin to function, the right-to-left ventricular shunt in the heart closes, and in certain species a peeping sound may be heard from the egg. At this time, turning of the egg should cease, and it is placed on the bottom of the incubator. Twitching of the abdominal muscles, which occurs secondary to breathing, causes the exteriorized yolk sac to be drawn into the chick's abdomen. With subsequent breaths, the level of CO_2 within the air cell rises. When CO_2 reaches 10%, the pipping muscle again begins to twitch, causing the egg tooth to penetrate the shell; this is called external pip. At this time, the eggs are moved out of the incubator and into the hatcher. The time between entering the air cell and external pipping may range from 3 hours to 3 days, but is typically 24 to 48 hours for most psittacine birds.[6]

Malposition and inadequate moisture loss are among the most common causes of embryonic mortality prior to hatching. Malpositions commonly occur secondary to hyperthermia or elevated temperatures, which also cause premature pipping. Two of the most common psittacine malpositions are when the head is located at the small end of the egg and when the beak is rotated away from the air cell. Eggs incubated below optimum temperatures develop slower and typically have increased problems with hatching. Excessive humidity fosters the development of "wet chicks." These chicks drown at pipping, due to remaining albumin, and are often edematous. Eggs exposed to low humidity may dry out, causing adherence of the shell membrane to the chick, preventing normal pipping.

All dead eggs should undergo necropsy by the avian veterinarian or aviculturist. During the gross necropsy, the embryo's general condition and position are assessed. Abnormal tissues and fluids are cultured and/or sent off for histopathologic examination. The shell is examined for color, texture, shape, and the presence or absence of stress lines. Thickness of the shell is assessed by differences in texture, as well as transparency and the degree of porosity.

NEONATAL CARE AND FEEDING

Once hatched, or pulled from the nest, neonatal or young chicks should be housed in warm appropriate environments such as forced air incubators like Lyon Technologies Animal Intensive Care Units (Lyon Technologies Inc, Chuls Vista, CA, USA). They should be on scheduled feeding as described later because nutrition is paramount to their survival.

Nutrition is also key during conception, incubation, and parental feeding of baby chicks. Parents must be fed nutritionally complete diets including large amounts of fresh fruits and vegetables plus breeder pelleted diets. Larger psittacines should also receive large nuts (hazelnuts, brazil nuts, macadamia nuts); medium psittacines should also receive smaller nuts (pine nuts, pistachios, almonds); and small psittacines should receive healthier seed choices such as safflower, rape, and flax seeds. Vitamin and mineral supplements should not be provided, with the exception of natural cuttlebone. Cuttlebone should be available for all breeding birds both large and small. Crush and serve it in the food bowls for larger breeding birds, and have it secured inside the cages with the soft side facing in for smaller breeding birds.

A healthy chick should have a healthy vigorous feeding response whether its parents or an owner is feeding it. The chick's feeding response is referred to as "pumping." If chicks do not pump, then their parents or an owner cannot safely feed them. Therefore, it will not matter how balanced and complete a diet you feed the parents or prepare for a chick, if the chick is not able to receive it safely into the crop.

Psittacine chicks do best on higher-fat diets, such as Kaytee Macaw Exact or Kaytee High Fat Hand Feeding Formula (Kaytee Products Inc, Chilton, WI, USA). Most psittacines do well on these types of diets, unless they are prone to obesity and hepatic lipidosis, like white and pink/salmon-colored cockatoos. The percentage of solids (the powdered formula) mixed should be 27%. Handfeeding formula should be mixed with clean, hot water. The temperature of the final formula mix should be between 105° and 108°F.

Temperatures lower than 105°F may result in formula aspiration, especially in Eclectus and African grey parrots, as chicks will not pump if the formula is not warm enough. This will result in aspiration and subsequent aspiration pneumonia. Temperatures of 109°F or higher or microwave reheating will result in crop burns. Microwave reheating causes crop burns because formula is a powder-and-liquid mixture. Unblended tiny amounts of powder can harbor heat, forming a closed ball of heat that explodes when it comes in contact with liquid in the crop, or beyond, in the bird's gastrointestinal tract. Crop burns can take up to 3 weeks to fistulate out of the body and, if not treated properly, can be fatal. If crop burns fistulate into the coelomic cavity, usually in the thoracic area, they are acutely fatal. Hence, it is best to never microwave any food at all for birds.

It is important to make sure handfeeding syringes be scrubbed clean, disinfected, and dried or discarded after every use. Hot soapy water wash, followed by soaking in diluted Roccal-D (Pfizer) and rinsing with a very dilute chlorhexidine mixture, works well. Every chick should have its own syringe for each feeding. Chicks should be fed on schedule or as soon as their crops are almost empty during the day. It is not necessary to feed chicks after midnight and before sunrise as they need to rest. Poor doers and sick or stunted chicks may need supplemental night feedings. Chicks should be weighed every morning before feeding, and their weights should be recorded, monitored, and compared to growth charts for the same species. Chicks must gain weight daily until weaning. A lack of weight gain or actual weight loss often indicates a problem is developing.

Chicks being handfed from day 1 require a diluted commercial formula for their first 3 days of life. These neonates should be started on a dilute commercial formula, such as Kaytee Macaw Exact, which should be fed until day 4. The macaw formulas are higher in fat and calcium and lower in vitamin D, all of which are important for healthy neonatal chick development. The diluted formula is given every 2 hours of the first and second days, except during the night, when crops are allowed to empty. On day 2, neonates should receive BENE-BAC PLUS Bird and Reptile (PetAg, Hampshire, IL, USA) (0.1 mL) at their first feeding. The third-day feedings are given every 3 hours.

By day 4, neonates should be started on an undiluted formula mixture. The schedule of formula feedings after day 3 goes from: 5 times a day for the smallest of birds, to 4 times a day, to 3 times, to 2 times, to 1 times, to weaning for birds of conure size and up. Birds are gradually moved down based on their species and individual size. The amounts fed are based on body weight (BW) early on, later by species (see later). Hence, on day 4, Kaytee Regular Exact is fed to all the white and pink/salmon-colored cockatoos. The cockatoos are fed at 10% BW until 3 times a day, when they are switched to 8% to prevent hepatic lipidosis. Birds that require more fat such as the black/gray cockatoos, thick-billed parrots, hyacinth macaws, green-winged macaws, golden conures, and slender-billed cockatoos do best when fed a macaw handfeeding formula with added fat and fiber (see description). The hyacinth macaws are fed such a formula at 12% BW and the green-winged macaws at 11%; all the other birds in this group are fed at 10% BW. The rest of the macaw species, African greys, Caiques, sun conures, Eclectus parrots, and hawk-headed parrots do best on the Kaytee Macaw Exact handfeeding formula. All these birds are fed at 10% BW, except for the Buffon's macaw, which is fed at 12% of BW. Once the birds reach their twice-a-day feeding, they are gradually increased to a once-a-day predetermined maximum for their species. For example, the maximum volume is 5 mL for cockatiels, 25 mL for sun conures, 50 mL for African greys, and 140 mL for hyacinth macaws.

At 2 feedings a day the juvenile birds should be offered solid foods, such as pellets (Zupreem Fruit Blend [Hill's Pet Nutrition, Inc., Topeka, KS, USA], Kaytee Rainbow Chunky [Keytee Products, Inc], LaFeber [Lafeber Company, Cornell, IL, USA]), fruits and vegetables, and shaved nut pieces or small nuts such as pine nuts. Vitamin and mineral supplements should not be provided. Be careful with larger pieces of fruits and nut treats with big macaws (eg, whole grapes and ¼ orange slices with the rinds on, etc). Such food items can be swallowed whole, causing crop impaction and gastrointestinal blockage.

Water bowls should be introduced when the birds are at 1 feeding a day. Once birds are drinking and eating on their own, they can be moved into larger cages or flights. Birds can be trained to use a drinking Lixit L-100 (an automated watering device; ATCO Manufacturing Company Inc) before their water bowls are removed as needed. Birds should always be weighed and monitored closely during the weaning process. Birds should never be force weaned. Instead, each should be treated as an individual and weaned at his or her own pace.

If baby birds are sold before they are weaned, intense avian veterinary help is needed. Unweaned baby birds continue to perpetuate the creation of special clients, and patients, who need extensive time commitments from their avian veterinarians. Such a service could never be achieved through office visit consultation alone. The methodical repetitive education of their new owners is the best way to help these baby birds.

PEDIATRIC HISTORY AND PHYSICAL EXAMINATION

Psittacine pediatric medicine is complex, the majority of complicating issues are management related, and the number one management issue is nutrition as described earlier. A thorough pediatric history and complete physical examination are a must.

Pediatric History

Note the parent's health and breeding history, the condition of chick's clutchmates and other siblings, and any problems the chick has and may have had during incubation and hatching. Bloodwork, other labwork, radiographs, and even a housecall visit may be necessary.

As part of the history, evaluate the chick's diet. Note the preparation, temperature, delivery, method of handfeeding, and hygiene, as well as the amount and frequency of feeding. Determine if feeders are washing their hands with a disinfectant soap before handling each chick and between groups of chicks.

Determine whether the bird's crop is empty before each feed, especially the first feed of the day. Assess environment, housing, and substrate for cleanliness, safety, and warmth. Inquire as to the behavior of the chick, its feeding response, and the color, consistency, and volume of its feces, urine, and urates.

Pediatric Physical Examination

The physical examination of the chick should entail evaluating weight charts for daily gain, assessing overall appearance, proportions, and behavior. In neonates, this exam should be performed in a warm room with prewarmed hands.[6,9–12] Knowledge of different species' growth rates, development, and behavioral characteristics are helpful.[12] Owners should examine each chick daily checking for potential problems. They should start from the tip of the beak and end at the toes. The beak should be straight and well aligned and monitored for malocclusion at each feeding.[13] The beak should also be warm. The mouth and tongue should be clean, dry, and free of mucus or plaque.[14] The crop should be soft, empty between feeds, and never pendulous. The legs should be straight and properly positioned. The feet should be warm and pointing forward. The skin should be light pink. The droppings should be moist and well formed with a small amount of white urates and urine. The chick should sleep between feedings and not beg incessantly.

Psittacine neonates are altricial.[6,9–12] Nourishment, warmth, food, and a safe environment must be provided. Neonatal chicks must be kept in an incubator with an air temperature of 93° to 98°F.[6,9–12] External heat must be provided until the chicks reach 1½ months of age. Smaller containers lined with white paper towels help prevent spraddle leg, keep each chick safe, and allow their droppings to be carefully monitored. After 1½ months chicks can be moved into plastic containers lined with white paper towels kept in warm enclosures with limited drafts, such as fish tanks. Warmth continues to be an issue, and, if the temperature falls, so may the growth rates, digestion, and viability of the chicks. Poor doers and sick or stunted chicks require higher temperatures than do healthy chicks of the same age. Although it is safest to house neonatal psittacines separately, heat is a bigger issue with solely housed chicks. Chicks housed with others are at risk of trauma issues when hungry babies pump on each other before or during scheduled feedings. Heat and humidity are issues for chicks of all ages; make sure that both are being provided. Older chicks can be kept on white towels so as to continue monitoring of their droppings. Wood shavings or crumbled paper substrates are dangerous for chicks of any age or health status, as they could be ingested. Chicks can also fall or burrow into crumbled paper substrates, causing potential suffocation, regurgitation, aspiration, and death.

In neonates, most abdominal organs can be seen through the skin. Neonates normally have a visible liver, duodenal loop, yolk sac, and ventriculus and occasionally lung. The lungs and heart should be auscultated. Assess body mass by palpation of elbows, toes, and hips, as keel muscle mass is not a reliable indicator of BW in the very young. Crops should be examined visually for size and color and carefully palpated for thickness, tone, burns, punctures, or the presence of foreign bodies. Crops should also be transilluminated to attempt to evaluate and describe their contents. Skin should be evaluated for color, texture, hydration, and the presence of subcutaneous fat. Normally, psittacine chicks should have beige-pink, warm, and supple skin (**Fig. 1**). Dehydration causes a chick's skin to become dry, hyperemic, and tacky (**Fig. 2**).

In juveniles, feathers should be examined for stress marks, color bars or shade changes, hemorrhage, or deformities of shafts and emerging feathers. The musculo-skeletal system should be palpated and assessed for skeletal defects or trauma in chicks of all ages. Until weaning, cockatoo chicks sit back on their hocks and are balanced forward on their large abdomens. Macaws prefer to lie down. Chicks normally have prominent abdomens, due to a food-filled crop, proventriculus, ventriculus, and small intestine. Beaks should be examined for malformations when

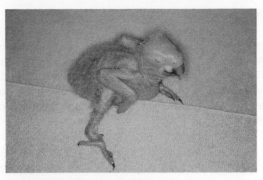

Fig. 1. Healthy plump well-hydrated macaw chick.

the bird's mouth is closed.[13] Pump pads (the soft fleshy part of the baby bird's beak at its commissures) should be examined for wounds and the feeding response elicited. Generally, a healthy baby bird should elicit a vigorous feeding response when stimulated at the beak's lateral commissures. The eyes and the periocular region should be examined for any abnormalities including lid defects, swelling, discharge, crusting, or blepharospasm. Normally a clear discharge is noted in the eyes when they are first opening, which typically occurs unilaterally. Eyes begin to open on days 14 to 28 for macaws, 10 to 21 for cockatoos, and 14 to 21 for Amazons. Nares and ears should be examined for discharge and aperture size or absence. The oral cavity should be examined for plaques, inflammation, or injuries.

If a baby bird dies, gross necropsies can be very informative and should be performed in all cases. Histopathology may lead to a definitive diagnosis facilitating proper preventative medical management of the original collection. With the pet owner's consent and permission, information gained can be relayed to the aviculturist. Based on this information, and the collection's general health history, you can better treat, and hence protect, the rest of the flock.

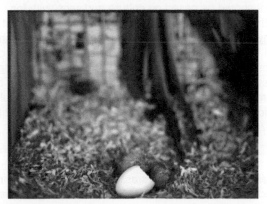

Fig. 2. Recently hatched blue and gold macaw chick. Note pink/red tacky dehydrated skin. Not plump, soft, light pink to beige and well hydrated.

Pediatric Diagnostics

Clinical pathology

Hematology and clinical chemistries should be performed by taking blood from the right jugular vein. As with adults, blood samples drawn should be less than 1% of the bird's BW. Toenail clips should be reserved for blood sexing only. Young chicks have lower packed cell volumes and lower total protein compared to adults. Their albumin and uric acid values are lower, and their alkaline phosphatase and creatine phosphokinase values are higher.

Microbiology

Cloacal culture, crop culture, fecal cytology, and Gram stain examinations should be performed during routine examination. Normally, cloacal and crop flora are gram positive and consist of *Lactobacillus, Corynebacteria, Staphlylococcus,* and nonhemolytic *Streptococcus.* Most gram-negative and anaerobic bacteria are considered pathogenic, as are yeast. Choanal cultures should be taken if upper respiratory tract disease is suspected or if choanal papillae are abnormally blunted.

Radiology

The crop, proventriculus, and ventriculus are normally enlarged in neonatal and juvenile birds pre-weaning, and the latter 2 take up much of the abdominal cavity on radiographs. Furthermore, muscle mass is reduced.

Endoscopy

Endoscopy, and surgery in general, is best performed on the fasted pediatric patient, since the proventriculus, ventriculus, and intestines are normally enlarged in unweaned birds. If the birds are kept warm and stable, anesthesia and endoscopy are quick. It is safest to scope after weaning, but the author has safely scoped much younger birds, birds being fed 3 times a day and less being the cutoff for endoscopy. If feeding occurs soon after recovery, then hypothermia, hypoglycemia, and hypocalcemia are easily avoidable. Endoscopy is useful for foreign body retrieval, syrinx examination, surgical sexing, and exploratory coelomic examination.

TREATMENT

Antimicrobials

Antibiotic treatment should be based on culture and sensitivity for 7 days. The author believes strongly that all pediatric patients on antibiotics should automatically be put on the antifungal nystatin. *Lactobacillus* supplementation is also highly recommended after antimicrobial treatment, at hatch, and 2 days after hatch. Mild yeast infections can be treated with nystatin alone for 14 days. Retractable yeast infections should be treated with the systemic antifungal ketoconazole (30 mg/kg) in combination with nystatin for a minimum of 21 days. Refractory yeast infections should also be treated with an acetic acid crop gavage (10 mL/kg) at the end of the antifungal treatment, followed by *Lactobacillus.*

Fluids

In pediatrics, patient stabilization centers around temperature and rehydration. Oral, subcutaneous, and intravascular fluids are all warmed and given as needed. Subcutaneous fluids are the most frequently used (100 mL/kg). In the severely dehydrated neonate, a jugular catheter is the preferred rehydration route.

COMMON PEDIATRIC PROBLEMS
Unretracted Yolk Sac

The yolk sac, a diverticulum of the small intestine, is normally internalized into the abdomen before hatching. It is absorbed over the next few days, providing the chick with nourishment and maternal antibodies. Retention of the yolk sac within the abdomen, another problem, commonly occurs secondary to *Escherichia coli* omphalitis. Unretracted yolk sacs can also occur secondary to infections but are typically a result of incubation problems, such as elevated incubation temperatures. Chicks with unretracted yolk sacs, and therefore an open umbilicus, should be placed on clean towels in the hatcher or the incubator, and their umbilicus swabbed with chlorhexidine scrub. Crop and cloacal cultures should be taken, as well as yolk sac cultures if the sac is leaking. The chicks should be placed on appropriate antibiotics and oral antifungals. Chicks should also be treated with fluids. If the yolk sac fails to become internalized, surgery is necessary.

Stunting

Stunting, commonly caused by malnutrition, is most pronounced in the first 30 days of life. Affected birds have poor growth rates, low weight, and an enlarged head relative to their body size. They also have thin legs and wings and abnormal feather growth including delayed emergence (on the body), misdirection (top of head), and feather stress or color bar lines. Stunted birds are typically poor doers, have crop stasis, and have red, wrinkled, and dehydrated skin. Possible causes of stunting include inadequate warmth, poor nutrition, poor formula preparation, poor and infrequent delivery of formula, and exposure to bacteria and/or fungus. Treatment is supportive and includes placing the chick in an incubator, frequent feeding of high fat formula such as Kaytee Macaw Exact, a crop bra, fluids, and antibiotics and antifungals as indicated by diagnostics.

Leg and Toe Deformities

Splay leg, a common deformity, is thought to occur secondary to malnutrition, obesity, improper substrate or enclosures, or a congenital defect. Once identified it should be treated immediately. Usually one leg is affected, but both can be. Juveniles that splay on pellets, or other slippery substrates, may straighten up on towels or packed towels. For best results, affected neonates should be packed in paper towels and/or hobbled. Simple hobbling may be sufficient. For severe cases, hobbling of both feet to a flat small plank, similar to a snowboard, so that the legs are properly positioned and the toes face forward may be necessary. Once both feet are hobbled and attached to the plank, the chick should be placed into a small straight-sided container (**Fig. 3**). For best results, hobbling of either kind must be changed frequently due to soiling and growth of the chick. If hobbling does not work, ostectomy may be indicated. Crooked, crossed, or forwardly directed toes can be corrected by splinting if caught early; otherwise, surgery may also be indicated.

Constricted Toes

Constricted toe syndrome, of unknown etiology, occurs most commonly in Eclectus, macaws, and gray parrots. The lesion consists of an annular ring constriction usually on the last phalanx and most frequently affecting the outer toes, numbers 1 and 4. Under isoflurane anesthesia and magnification, rule out cloth or other fibers as a cause. Next, debride the circumferential fibrotic annular band with fine forceps. Finally, put 2 full-thickness longitudinal incisions, medially and laterally, through the

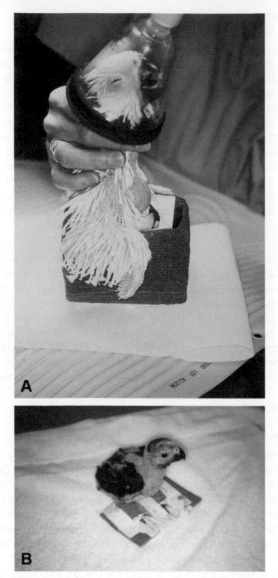

Fig. 3. (*A*) Board-hobbled umbrella cockatoo baby. (*B*) Board-hobbled African grey baby.

constriction band, express accumulated serum, bandage, and monitor for swelling. Soak in warm dilute chlorhexadine solution and massage daily, then re-bandage. Chicks should be cloacal and crop cultured and put on parenteral antibiotics and oral antifungals.

Beak Malformations

The 3 most common beak malformations are lateral deviations of the maxilla (scissor beak) (**Fig. 4**), mandibular compression deformities of the mandible, and prognathism (pug beak) (**Fig. 5**). Lateral deviation is thought to be congenital or induced by poor handfeeding technique. Mandibular compression is thought to be

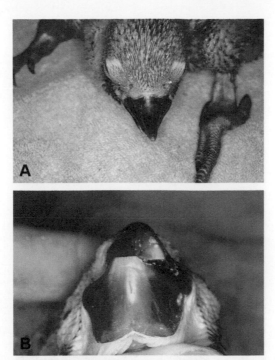

Fig. 4. (*A*) Scissor beak in a Canindae juvenile macaw, dorsal view. (*B*) Scissor beak in a Canindae juvenile macaw, ventral view.

induced by rough handfeeding technique. Prognathism (pug beak) is thought to be congenital. The first 2 malformations are most common in macaws, while the third is most common in cockatoos. When the chicks are young and the beaks are most pliable, physical therapy and trimming are indicated. After calcification, frequent trimming, acrylic implants, or extensions are often needed to correct the malformations.

Regurgitation

During weaning, the crop normally shrinks in size. Hence, regurgitation of small amounts of food post-feeding signals the need to reduce the frequency of feedings and begin introducing solid foods such as pellets, fruits, and vegetables. Typically, as a bird grows, feeding volumes are increased and the frequency of feeds is decreased. Younger birds will regurgitate if overfed and this can lead to aspiration pneumonia. Repeated regurgitation in a chick that is too young to wean or regurgitation of large volumes may indicate disease or mechanical blockage. Rule out foreign bodies, crop or lower gastrointestinal fungal or bacterial infection, gout, or proventricular dilatation disease. Drugs such as trimethoprim-sulfa, doxycycline, and nystatin can cause regurgitation, especially in macaw chicks. Chicks should be worked-up and started on antibiotics and antifungals as needed. Note that in cases of regurgitation, antibiotics should be given parentally.

Esophagitis or Pharyngitis

Infections of the esophagus and/or pharynx clinically manifest as ulcers and white, gray, or yellow plaques in the mouth. Thick oral mucus is common in these cases, and

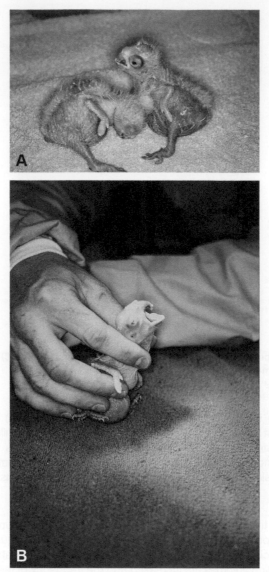

Fig. 5. (*A*) Prognathic beak in umbrella cockatoo baby. (*B*) Prognathic beak in umbrella cockatoo baby.

food and debris may accumulate inside and around the mouth, beak, and tongue. Common causes include gram-negative bacterial and yeast infections from unclean formula or water and its delivery. Antibiotics and antifungals should be given orally. Fluids can be given subcutaneously.

Esophageal or Pharyngeal Punctures

Esophageal or pharyngeal punctures occur secondary to syringe or tube feeding. They are most common in vigorously pumping birds, like macaws. Esophageal punctures usually occur midway between the pharynx and the thoracic inlet in the cranialmost aspect of the crop. Pharyngeal punctures usually occur in the caudal aspect of the pharynx slightly caudal to the right of the glottis. Emergency surgery is needed to remove subcutaneously deposited food, create a drain, and begin flushing of the wound. The bird must be tube fed directly into the crop so food does not come in contact with the wound during healing. The crop, cloaca, and choana should be cultured, a complete blood count and chemistry submitted, and the bird started on antibiotics and antifungals.

Crop Stasis

Crop stasis is very common in neonatal and juvenile birds. Primary causes of crop stasis include infection, crop foreign bodies, atony, burns, dehydration of food in the crop, hypothermia, formula that is too cold or too hot, and inappropriate environmental temperature. Some of the most common foreign bodies include feeding tubes, syringe tips, or bedding material such as shavings. The most common primary cause of crop stasis is yeast or candidiasis. Secondary causes include distal gut stasis due to ileus, intestinal intussusception, bacterial or fungal infection, sepsis, dilation, proventricular dilatation disease, polyomavirus, gastrointestinal foreign bodies, and renal or hepatic failure. Medical and mechanical management are typically needed for the treatment of crop stasis. Treatment includes placing the chick in a warm incubator with oxygen as needed. Crop washing with warm saline and chlorhexidine, after cultures are performed, is done to empty the pendulous crop. Small, frequent gavage feedings along with appropriate antibiotic and antifungal treatment are appropriate. Finally, the chick should be fitted with a crop bra, which is only released during feedings. Diagnostics as described earlier are very important, especially culture, crop and fecal cytology, and bloodwork. Further diagnostics, such as radiography, crop biopsy, and/or reduction, should be performed as needed. Fluids are key in the treatment of both crop and other gastrointestinal tract stasis cases. Oral fluids rehydrate inspissated crop material and hasten its passage. Subcutaneous fluids are the treatment of choice for systemic rehydration (100 mL/kg). Intravenus fluids are best in a severely dehydrated moribund patient. In these cases, placement of a right jugular intravenous catheter is preferred; these catheters are safely maintained for days. If the crop is severely impacted, repeated flushing with warm saline may be needed to empty it. The crop bra mentioned is a simple form of mechanical management for the overstretched crop. The bras are made in-house of VetWrap (3M Animal Care Products, St Paul, MN, USA; a large cross of VetWrap is fit with a horizontal rectangular piece of VetWrap placed where the strips crosses over (**Fig. 6**). In a severely overstretched crop, reduction surgery may be necessary to facilitate emptying. Further, hypoproteinemia may occur secondary to severe chronic crop stasis. In these cases, whole blood transfusions and metoclopromide or cisapride may be indicated, as long as gastrointestinal obstruction has been ruled out.

Chronic nonresponsive crop stasis may involve mural candidiasis. These cases are best diagnosed with biopsy and require long-term systemic antifungal and antibiotic treatment and acetic acid gavage. Acetic acid acidifies the crop's contents and discourages yeast and bacterial growth. The most common clinical signs of crop stasis are a visibly oversized static crop and regurgitation. Although a manageable problem, crop stasis can be a fatal condition due to dehydration and sepsis and, therefore, demands immediate intervention. Crop stasis, the most common pediatric problem, causes dehydration. Sepsis typically follows dehydration, and together these conditions are the most common killers in avian pediatrics.

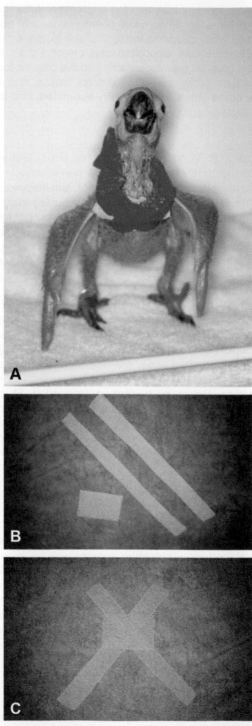

Fig. 6. (*A*) Slightly thin and dehydrated macaw chick with crop bra. (*B*) Crop bra preparation strip. (*C*) Crop bra cross strips.

Crop Burns

Crop burns of the mucosa and skin occur secondary to feeding excessively hot food ($\geq$109°F). The burn must fistulate through and out of the body before surgery and this may take weeks. Clinical signs of crop burn before fistulation include a poor appetite, swelling and discoloration of the neck or crop, and weight loss. If the crop fistulates, a visible scab forms over the burned area, which when ruptured allows food to pour out of the body. If the crop fistulates into the body or coelomic cavity or between the skin and the crop, the event is most often fatal. Step 1 to a fistulated crop repair is aggressive surgical removal of the burned tissue and scab. Next, the skin and the crop tissues need to be delicately separated and closed in separate layers. An inverting pattern may be used on the crop itself. Antibiotics and antifungals are necessary, both before and after surgery. A common mistake is to attempt a surgical repair too early. Trying to remove and close the burned tissue before all the damaged tissue has become evident may result in incorporating damaged tissue into the repair. This will dehisce as further necrosis occurs and requires another surgery.

Foreign Body Ingestion or Impaction

Neonates and juveniles are curious and will ingest foreign bodies, if available. If large and within the crop, foreign bodies can be removed via retrograde palpation and a finger swipe or carefully with long hemostats. Alligator hemostats can be especially useful. A ingluvotomy may be required to remove any material that cannot be removed via the esophagus. Smaller pieces, such as wood shavings, may pass through the crop and result in lower gastrointestinal impactions. Emergency surgery is often indicated.

LESS COMMON PEDIATRIC PROBLEMS
Rectal Prolapse

Secondary to hypermotility or infection, rectal prolapse has been reported in macaws. If the prolapse is fresh, the tissue may be salvaged. Emergency surgery is indicated.

Intestinal Intussusception

Intestinal intussusceptions have been noted by the author in juvenile Amazons, but could occur in any species. Bloodwork and cultures should be taken. Birds should be started on antibiotics and antifungals. Emergency surgery is often indicated; however, the prognosis is grave.

Hepatic Hematomas

These are suspected to be secondary to rough handling/trauma or possibly dietary deficiencies. Most reports have been in macaws where the etiology is unknown. Bloodwork and cultures should be taken; chicks should be started on vitamin K1 and given transfusions as needed.

Hepatic Lipidosis

Hepatic lipidosis occurs secondary to overfeeding calories or genetic predisposition primarily in handfed umbrella cockatoos, Moluccan cockatoos, and blue-and-gold macaws, but it can occur in other birds.

Affected chicks have severely enlarged livers visible through the skin and enlarged abdomens and may be pale and dyspnic. These birds need to have their intake per-feeding reduced and their frequency of feedings increased immediately to help decrease their dyspnea. Their dietary fat content needs to be reduced. Bloodwork and cultures should be taken, and the birds should be started on milk thistle and lactulose.

Gout

Gout, a clinical sign, occurs secondary to severe renal disease and severe dehydration. In juvenile macaws, gout is thought to occur secondary to excess vitamin D_3 and calcium in the diet. In blue and gold macaws, red fronted macaws, cockatiels, and palm cockatoos, a genetic predisposition is suspected.

Wine-Colored Urine

Wine-colored urine may occur in juvenile African grey, Amazon, and pionus parrots. It may occur secondary to certain handfeeding formulas and is most obvious on white or light-colored towels.

DISEASES IN THE NURSERY
Polyomavirus

Polyomavirus is the most common viral disease encountered in psittacine nurseries. It is highly contagious, has an estimated incubation period of 2 weeks, and is typically widespread before detection. Most affected birds die within 24 to 48 hours. Hence, it is an acute and rapidly fatal disease of hand-raised neonates. Two- to 14-week-old macaws, conures, Eclectus, and ring-necks are most commonly affected. If clinical signs appear at all, they consist of weakness, pallor, subcutaneous hemorrhage, anorexia, dehydration, crop stasis, regurgitation, vomiting, and depression. Hemorrhage is noted at injection sites, plucked feathers bleed excessively, and petechial and ecchymotic hemorrhages appear on the skin. Survivors exhibit poor weight gain, polyuria, gut stasis, and abnormal feathering similar to that seen with psittacine beak and feather disease (PBFD). Asymptomatic infection keeps this virus in the psittacine population. A DNA polyoma cloacal swab test is available to identify actively shedding birds. Thus, the best method to manage polyoma virus is by vaccination with the killed polyoma vaccine manufactured by Biomune (Psittimune APV; Bioimune Co, Lenexa, KS, USA). The entire aviary and all the chicks in the nursery should be vaccinated. Strict nursery husbandry and a closed nursery policy (including showering in) should also be practiced. Biosecurity is the best prevention.

Proventricular Dilatation Disease

This is also an important viral disease of the pediatric patient. Affected birds range from 10 weeks and up and the disease may be fatal. In the nursery, chicks may exhibit regurgitation, crop stasis, voluminous feces, weight loss, weakness, and neurologic signs, including head tremors. Biopsy of the ventriculus, the proventriculus, or the crop may be diagnostic, when lymphocytic plasmocytic infiltrates of myenteric plexi are noted. A closed nursery and strict biosecurity are the best tools available to control this virus.

Psittacine Beak and Feather Disease

PBFD can occur in neonates, is highly contagious, and is easily spread by feather dust and dander. This viral disease is characterized by pterylodysplasia (abnormal feather growth) and is most often noted in fully feathered chicks. Feathers can be clubbed and can have circumferential constrictions, and sheaths and blood feathers may be retained. A DNA PBFD whole blood test is available to identify positive birds. Positive birds should be isolated and retested in 90 days as some may clear the virus. The disease course may be acute or chronic depending on the age and immunocompetence of the individual. The entire aviary should be tested for PBFD, and positive adult birds should be immediately removed from the collection. Strict nursery husbandry and quarantine should be practiced, and all chicks should be tested before leaving the nursery.

Poxvirus

This virus can be problematic in neotropical collections where chicks remain in the nest for any length of time or where juveniles are housed outdoors.

Microbial Infections

Microbial alimentary infections are among the most common problems in psittacine chicks. They are typically diagnosed by cloacal and crop cultures and gram stains. Gram-negative bacteria or yeast infections are abnormal in psittacine chicks. Some strains of E coli, Klebsiella spp, and Enterobacter spp are thought to vary in pathogenicity and can be isolated from completely normal chicks. Birds should be treated only if they exhibit clinical signs or if gram-negative bacteria or yeast are identified in large numbers. Further, they should only be treated based on culture and sensitivity. As mentioned earlier, all pediatric patients put on antibiotics must be put on the antifungal nystatin. In cases of regurgitation or stasis, antibiotics should be given subcutaneously until crop emptying or stasis improves. Microbial diseases of importance in the nursery include E coli spp, Klebsiella spp, Enterobacter spp, Pseudomonas spp, Salmonella spp, and Candida spp.

Chlamydophilia

Chlamydophilia should be screened for in all cases of nursery mortality, especially if the collection contains budgerigars or cockatiels. Unfortunately, the diagnosis of Chlamydophilia is difficult, and culture and isolation comprise the only definitive test. Chlamydophilia-positive birds must be treated with doxycycline for 45 days. The zoonotic potential of this disease must be discussed with the owners and reported to the health department if indicated.

ACKNOWLEDGMENTS

The author would like to thank Dr Paul McCurdy and Lisa Smith, CVT for their expert advice and opinion on this article.

REFERENCES

1. Romagnano A. Aviary design and management. In: Ballard B, Cheek R, editors. Exotic animal medicine for the veterinary technician. 2nd edition. Ames (IA): Wiley-Blackwell; 2010. p. 55–60.
2. Romagnano A, Hadley T. Sex differentiation and reproduction. In: Ballard B, Cheek R, editors. Exotic animal medicine for the veterinary technician. 2nd edition. Ames (IA): Wiley-Blackwell; 2010. p. 61–5.
3. Valentine M. Chromosomal analysis. In: Abramson J, Speer B, Thomsen J, editors. The large macaws: their care, breeding and conservation. Fort Bragg (NC): Raintree Publications; 1995. p. 73–7.
4. Clubb K, Swigert T. Commonsense incubation. In: Schubot RM, Clubb SL, Clubb KJ, editors. Psittacine aviculture: perspectives, techniques, and research. Loxahatchee (FL): Avicultural Breeding and Research Center; 1992. p. 9.1–15.1.

5. Clubb SL, Phillips A. Psittacine embryonic mortality. In: Schubot RM, Clubb SL, Clubb KJ, editors. Psittacine aviculture: perspectives, techniques, and research. Loxahatchee (FL): Avicultural Breeding and Research Center; 1992. p. 1–9.

6. Romagnano A. Reproduction and pediatrics. In: BSAVA manual of psittacine birds. 2nd edition. New York: Harcourt-Brown; 2005.

7. Clubb S. Psittacine pediatric husbandry and medicine. In: Altman RB, Clubb SL, Dorrestein GM, et al, editors. Avian medicine and surgery. Philadelphia: WB Saunders; 1997. p. 73–95.

8. Martin S, Romagnano A. Nest box preferences. In: Leusher A, editor. Parrot behavior. Ames (IA): Blackwell Publishing; 2006. p. 79–82.

9. Flammer K, Clubb S. Neonatology. In: Ritchie BW, Harrison GJ, Harrison LR, editors. Avian medicine: principles and application. Lake Worth (FL): Wingers; 1994. p. 805–38.

10. Clubb SL, Clubb KJ, Skidmore D, et al. Psittacine neonatal care and hand-feeding. In: Schubot RM, Clubb SL, Clubb KJ, editors. Psittacine aviculture: perspectives, techniques, and research. Loxahatchee (FL): Avicultural Breeding and Research Center; 1992. p. 11.1–12.1.

11. Phillips A, Clubb SL. Psittacine neonatal development. In: Schubot RM, Clubb SL, Clubb KJ, editors. Psittacine aviculture: perspectives, techniques, and research. Loxahatchee (FL): Avicultural Breeding and Research Center; 1992. p. 12.1–26.1.

12. Clubb KJ, Skidmore D, Schubot RM, et al. Growth rates of handfed psittacine chicks. In: Schubot RM, Clubb SL, Clubb KJ, editors. Psittacine aviculture: perspectives, techniques, and research. Loxahatchee (FL): Avicultural Breeding and Research Center; 1992. p. 14.1–19.1.

13. Wolf S, Clubb SL. Clinical management of beak malformations in handfed psittacine chicks. In: Schubot RM, Clubb SL, Clubb KJ, editors. Psittacine aviculture: perspectives, techniques, and research. Loxahatchee (FL): Avicultural Breeding and Research Center; 1992. p. 17.1-12.1.

14. Romagnano A. Examination and preventive medicine protocols in psittacines. In: Orcutt C, editor. Avian medicine. The Clinics Collection, Veterinary Clinics of North America, Exotic Animal Practice, Avian Pet Medicine. Saunders; 2005. p. 35–50.

Toucan Hand Feeding and Nestling Growth

Judy St. Leger, DVM, DACVP[a],*, Martin Vince, BS[b],
Jerry Jennings, BS, MBA[c], Erin McKerney, DVM[d], Erika Nilson, BS[a]

KEYWORDS
- Toucan • Toucanet • Aracari • Hand feeding
- Growth curve

Toucans and toucanets are charismatic ambassadors for the rainforest. Their presence in captive collections typifies the "jungle." Because of this, they are popular additions to aviaries in zoos and private avian collections. They are kept as pet birds but much less commonly than psittacines. When they are part of a pet bird collection, they are often included in small breeding programs.

Investigations to improve breeding and rearing programs remain to be performed for most toucan species. Elements of importance in captive propagation include adult management, nutrition, nest management, and egg/chick management. Variations in chick management and nutrition often result in variable fledging success between facilities. Small numbers of chicks for each facility make conducting large scale investigations impossible. Additionally, species-based variations and external factors such as clutch size impact both chick rearing success and growth. Objective criteria to gauge hand-rearing protocols are often limited to the number of birds raised to fledging. While this is a reasonable measure of success, information on chick development is helpful in determining effective hand feeding and chick health.

Toucans, toucanets, and aracaris all belong to the phylogenetic family Rhamphastidae. It is common to refer to this family as toucans. This is a large family consisting of 6 genera with 42 species. These birds occur over a large geographic area from southeastern Mexico extending into South America. Toucan habitat varieties range from forest lowland to mountain regions with birds residing at altitudes of 150 to 3600 m above sea level. As the biomes vary, so do diet and life history characteristics. In short, not all toucans are alike.[1]

Approximately 30 toucan species are currently found in captivity. Of these, reproductive success has been reported in at least 20. Rhamphastids can do an

The authors have nothing to disclose.

[a] SeaWorld San Diego, 500 SeaWorld Drive, San Diego, CA 92109, USA
[b] Riverbanks Zoo and Garden, PO Box 1060, Columbia, SC 29202, USA
[c] Emerald Forest Bird Garden, 38420 Dos Cameos Drive, Fallbrook, CA 92028, USA
[d] Peninsula Equine Medical Center, 100 Ansel Lane, Menlo Park, CA 94028, USA
* Corresponding author.
E-mail address: Judy.St.leger@seaworld.com

excellent job rearing their young with minimal intervention. However, hand feeding allows for control of early chick development and can be used to increase productivity. Artificial incubation can improve hatchability by reducing issues of egg damage or neglect from parents. Incubation results in a need to hand rear babies. To facilitate hand feeding, a retrospective study was performed to review hand-rearing considerations and develop growth curves for toucans. This information should serve as a guide to those looking to advance toucan aviculture.

MATERIALS AND METHODS

Hand feeding records and chick weights were obtained from Riverbanks Zoo (RBZ), Dallas World Aquarium (DWA), and Emerald Forest Bird Gardens (EFBG). These facilities represent 2 members of the Asociation of Zoos and Aquariums (AZA) and 1 private facility with a broad base of experience in hand rearing of toucans and toucanets. Over the past 20 years, these facilities have been the major producers of hand-reared rhamphastids in North America.

General information related to hand feeding was recorded for each facility. Specifics for incubation, brooding, hand feeding, and weaning were collected from 2 of the 3 facilities (RBZ and EFBG). Data collected from these 2 facilities include general incubation parameters, brooder temperatures and chick containment, and specifics about hand-feeding formulas and techniques.

Weight data from individual birds at all 3 facilities were tabulated for the first 60 days of life. Only species with growth data from more than 5 birds and more than 2 clutches were included in the production of growth curves. Data were not partitioned by facility or sex of the chicks. In total, data from 152 birds were used for development of the 8 growth curves. The legend for each curve indicates the number of birds and number of facilities used for curve development. Hand rearing for each species did not occur in every facility; keel bill toucan, collared aracari, and emerald toucanet data were each derived from only 1 facility. Data for all other species were derived from combined data from 2 facilities. No species was hand reared in all 3 facilities at levels that permitted aggregation of data from all participants.

Incubation schemes varied from fully parent incubated to fully artificially incubated. Many eggs that hatched in incubators spent between 1 and 7 days incubating under the parents. Determination of when to pull eggs was often based on past performance of the parental pair as well as management considerations like weather conditions and ease of incubation. Both parent-incubated and incubator-raised birds were used in curve development.

Nest-hatched birds were generally pulled for hand rearing between days 1 and 9. Fifty-nine nest-hatched birds (8 saffron, 8 Guyana, 1 chestnut-eared, 7 green aracari, 4 collared, 12 emerald, 12 toco, and 7 keel-billed) were included in this study. Weights were not measured on these chicks while they were under the care of parents in the nest. For those birds, daily weights were only considered during the hand-feeding period.

RESULTS
Incubation and Brooding

Incubation was reviewed for RBZ and EFBG. Incubation lengths vary but, in general, smaller birds such as toucanets and aracaris have a 16-day incubation period. Larger toucans such as the keel bills and tocos have a 16- to 18-day incubation. Regardless of whether chicks are reared by hand or by adults, juveniles are self-sufficient at or before 60 days of age. Many species demonstrate fledging at approximately 42 days. Artificial incubation techniques varied by facility and by

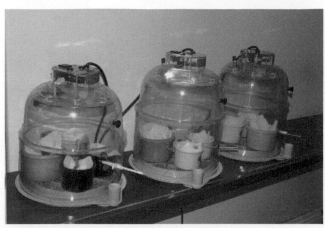

Fig. 1. Three brooder set-ups. Thermometers at the side measure temperature. Humidity is maximized with the ring at the bottom of the unit. Each cup contains 1 or 2 young chicks. (*Photograph courtesy of* Jerry Jennings, Fallbrook, CA.)

species. Incubation parameters include a high-quality incubator maintained at 98.5° to 99°F (36.9°–37.2°C) with a relative humidity maintained at 65%. Regular egg weights during incubation from EFBG were not available for review. RBZ maintains incubators such that eggs lose between 12% and 16% of its freshly laid weight during incubation. The relative humidity needed to achieve this may range from 65% to 95%, depending on factors such as eggshell quality. EFBG uses Turn-X incubators (Lyon Technologies, Chula Vista, CA, USA); eggs are automatically rotated using pans with a turning ring. RBZ uses Grumbach "Compact S84" incubators (Asslar, Germany); rollers turn the eggs hourly.

Brooder facilities at EFBG consist of temperature- and humidity-controlled containers (**Fig. 1**). Chicks are generally segregated by clutch. As the chicks grow, they are kept in larger containers or separated into individual containers. Brooder temperatures start at 97°F with relative humidity maintained at 93% to 95%. As chicks develop feathers and increase in size, brooder temperatures are decreased to ensure the comfort of the chicks. By day 7, brooders are maintained at 93° to 95° F for all infants. Chicks are held in bowls or cups with paper towels or towelling that is free of loose strings to ensure good footing and safety from tangles. Paper towels with 2-inch × 2-inch Rubbermaid (Atlanta, GA, USA) shelf liner on top are considered superior bedding at EFBG due to the ability for staff to easily assess the droppings.

Once feathered, baby toucans become much more active. Birds are moved from bowls to plastic tubs on absorbent wood pulp bedding (Carefresh by Absorption Corp., Ferndale, WA, USA). Development is rapid and impressive (**Fig. 2**). At approximately 6 weeks of age, most toucan species begin to fledge. Due to increased mobility at this phase of development, they are placed in weaning cages. These cages are equipped with 2 perches placed close to the bottom, to permit access to food bowls without the birds leaving the perch. Access to perches of the appropriate diameter is important. It can help prevent significant foot problems that may result from spending too long in a bowl or a cup. In nature young toucans exercise their feet for several days as they climb up and down the interior of the cavity to look out of the nest hole and prepare for fledging.

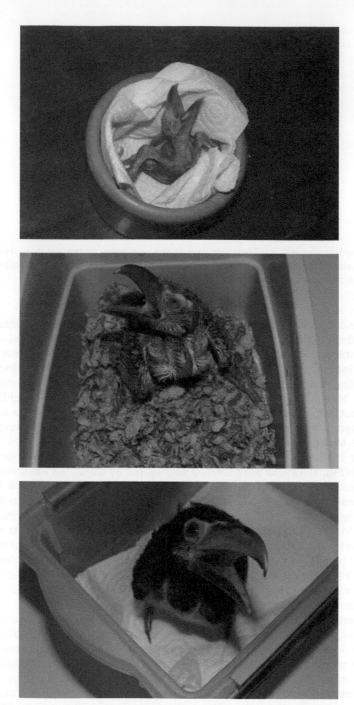

Fig. 2. Collared aracari (*Pteroglossus torquatus*) at 25 days in an individual bowl; at 30 days on wood pulp bedding in a tub; and at 45 days in a tub for feeding (birds at this age are transferred to a weaning cage to facilitate perching and self-feeding). (*Photograph courtesy of* Jerry Jennings, Fallbrook, CA.)

Hand feeding continues at 5 feedings per day. Four of the 5 feedings consist of formula; 1 consists of pieces of fruit and soaked pellets (Mazuri [A division of Purina Mills, Gray Summit, MO, USA] Low Iron Softbill pellets) offered by hand or with forceps. Over the next 2 to 3 weeks, babies begin to eat fruit and soaked pellets. The extent of self-feeding is gauged by monitoring their feces, which increasingly contain fruit and are the color of pellets. As the birds learn to feed themselves, they increasingly resist hand feeding. The number of hand feeding events is reduced to 3 times daily and then twice daily. Once they are weaned, the soaked pellets are gradually switched over to dry pellets. If the birds initially refuse dry pellets, they are offered soaked pellets until they accept the dry.

Hand Feeding

Ramphastids are eager eaters; they will gape at the slightest change in ambient light, nearby movement, and/or gentle tapping on the beak. They do not possess a crop, and thus hand feeding time is prolonged compared to hand feeding psittacines of comparable size. A 2- to 3-week bird can take as long as 30 minutes to feed as opposed to less than 5 minutes for a psittacine. The bird is full when the soliciting ends and the bird's head goes back as if satiated. Some birds will solicit even when fully fed. Both RBZ and EFBG feed formula that is prepared fresh for each feed. EFBG feeds formula that is at room temperature (80°–85°F); RBZ feeds formula at a temperature that is very warm to the touch (104°–106°F). EFBG uses disposable syringes and cups for the first 2 to 3 weeks of a bird's life. Both facilities clean syringes and supplies between each feeding and soak them in Nolvasan (Fort Dodge Animal Health, Fort Dodge, IA, USA) solution and rinse equipment before use.

EFBG uses Mazuri commercial hand feeding formula (Mazuri Hand Feeding Formula 5TMX) mixed with distilled water to a consistency of pea soup. To this, pureed commercial canned baby fruit is added at a ratio of 5% to 10% fruit to formula. The formula is fed by syringe based on the bird's body weight. Initial feeding are no more than 5% of the bird's body weight (total daily amount) for the first few days. The amount fed is increased over the hand rearing period based on the bird's increasing body weight and an increasing food amount such that by 6 weeks of age, birds are receiving 9% to 10% of body weight for total daily feeding.

At 6 hours post hatch, hand feeding begins with distilled water. Birds are given water at 25% of their body weight. At 12 hours they receive 25% of their body weight in half-strength formula such that an 8- to 10-g bird receives 0.2 mL of food in increments of 0.1 mL. Babies pulled from their parents are first fed 4 hours after their removal from the nest. For the first 3 weeks of life, babies are fed 9 times per day at 2-hour intervals from 6:00 AM through 6:00 PM, then at 8:30 PM and 11:30 PM. This schedule allows for maximum daily weight gain with a 6½-hour interval between the last and first feedings. Adding a 10th feeding does not improve weight gains.

Hand-feeding protocols for facility RBZ are similar with a few significant changes. Chicks are kept on a towel surface in a small dish at 99.0°F (37.2°C). Small feedings are given every 1.5 to 2 hours from about 7:00 AM 11:00 PM. As the chick grows, the time between feeds is increased along with the amount per feed; the chick is not fed through the night. A 1-mL syringe is used to feed young toucan chicks. Kaytee (Chilton, WI, USA) Exact Original Formula is used as the basic hand feeding product for this facility. The first feed is distilled water or an oral electrolyte such as Pedialyte (Abbott Laboratories, Columbus, OH, USA) with only a very light sprinkle of Kaytee. For all of the other feeds, the hand feeding formula is prepared, (and progressively thickened) according to the manufacturer's instructions. As is done at EFBG, pureed commercial canned baby food is added at a ratio of 5% to 10% fruit to formula.

The chick is weighed daily prior to feeding at the same time each day. After each feed, food residue is cleaned from chick's mouth with a small piece of moistened cloth or a cotton-tipped applicator. Once the chick is 7 or 8 days old, a transition from the liquid diet to the adult diet is made. Very small pieces of pinkie mice, soaked Hills Science Diet Canine kibble (Topeka, KS, USA), fruit and soaked pellets are fed. The pellets are Marion Zoological (Plymouth, MN, USA), Red Apple Jungle; they are moistened by soaking for 45 seconds in distilled water. The same brand of pellet is fed to the adults.

Medications

Both facilities administer oral Nystatin for the first 1 to 4 weeks of the chicks' life. EFBG has a regular administration frequency of 3 times daily for 1 to 4 weeks depending on the chick's general condition and growth. RBZ has a decreasing frequency for 3 weeks. Dosing starts at 3 times a day for the first week; twice a day for the second week; and finally once a day for the third week. RZP uses no medications when hand feeding chicks that are removed from the parents at 10 days of age or greater.

Weight Curves

All 3 facilities contributed to the development of growth curves for the 8 toucan species. The growth curves for each species are presented in **Figs. 3–6**. All curves detail weight changes from day 1 to day 60. In all species examined, early growth was completed by this age. Growth curves generally level off between days 34 and 40. Smaller species are generally self-sufficient by 45 days of age. Larger species such as toco and keel-billed toucans are self-sufficient at or before 60 days of age.

Fig. 3 illustrates the growth data for the keel bill and toco toucans. The keel bill curve was derived from data from 24 birds held in one facility and raised over a 5-year period. The toco toucan curve represents 20 birds from 2 facilities raised over a 4-year period. **Fig. 4** illustrates data from collared and green aracaris. The collared aracari curve is derived from data from 24 birds raised in 1 facility over 4 years. The green aracari data are based on data from 2 facilities raising 12 birds over the course of 3 years. **Fig. 5** depicts the data from chestnut-eared aracaris and saffron toucanets. Five birds from 2 facilities were available to produce the chestnut-eared curve. Two facilities and a total of 24 birds were examined for the production of the saffron toucanet growth curve. **Fig. 6** contains the growth curves for Guyana and emerald toucanets. Eight birds from 2 facilities and 35 birds from 1 facility were used to produce the respective graphs.

The curves all follow the path expected lag, log, and plateau growth phases. The components of growth can be characterized as a lag phase occurring from days 0 to approximately 10, a log phase of remarkable growth generally occurring from days 10 to 38, and a plateau phase extending from the late 30s to early 40s until day 60.

DISCUSSION

The goal of this investigation was to briefly review results of 3 strong toucan rearing programs as a foundation for other toucan rearing programs. The growth curves provide a template for aviculturalists and veterinarians in gauging individual development of hand-fed toucans. While individual birds may vary along the curve, these data are critical for determining whether growth rates are within a normal range for birds. Over time, it is expected that individual facilities will be able to generate their own growth curves based on their specific management programs.

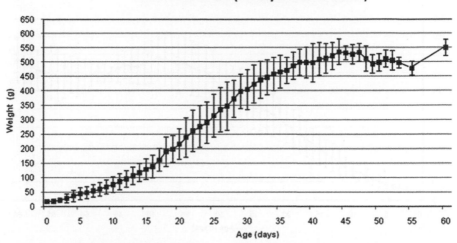

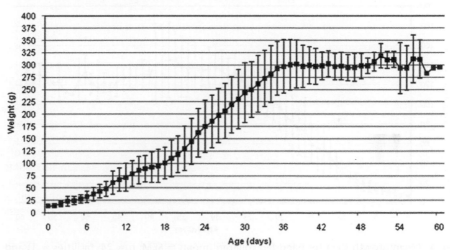

Fig. 3. Mean growth data for hand-fed toco (mean ± SEM; n = 20, facilities = 2) and keel-billed (mean ± SEM; n = 24, facilities = 1) toucans over the first 60 days of life.

The RBZ has led the zoo community in publishing data on toucan management, reproduction, and rearing. A good review of their hand-rearing efforts is available through the AZA *Toucan Husbandry Manual*.[2] Many of the features of the incubation and handrearing programs are equivelent to those used in psittacine rearing.[3,4] It is the nuances such as a modified feeding style that are critical to effective rearing of toucans compared to parrots. It is defining the differences in an objective manner that is needed to improve toucan hand rearing. All 3 facilities keep detailed notes on incubation and hand rearing. Further evaluations of these programs and their success and failures will be important in advancing aviculture.

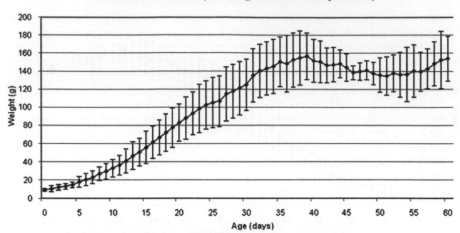

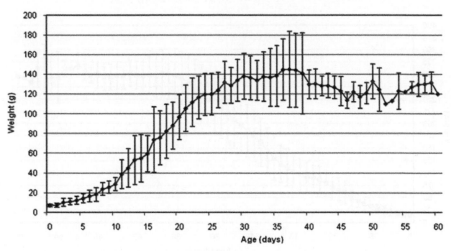

Fig. 4. Mean growth data for hand-fed collared (mean ± SEM; n = 24, facilities = 1) and green (mean ± SEM; n = 12, facilities = 2) aracaris over the first 60 days of life.

A variety of parameters were not specifically partitioned while deriving the growth curves. Sex determination was not available for many of the birds. Because of this, and because of the limited numbers of total birds, sex differences were not considered. It is likely that growth of chicks in the nestling phase is minimally impacted by chick sex. Facility differences in chick management and hand-feeding formulas were not considered in curve development. It is likely that this did impact the curves. However, by giving each facility an equal contribution based on chick production numbers and creating a weight band, it is hoped that the band realistically reflects expected fluxuations in chick weights. This band represents expected weights for chicks of the 8 species 95% of the time. Developing a band of expected chick weights is recognized as an effective way to create

Chestnut-eared Aracari (*Pteroglossus castanotis*)

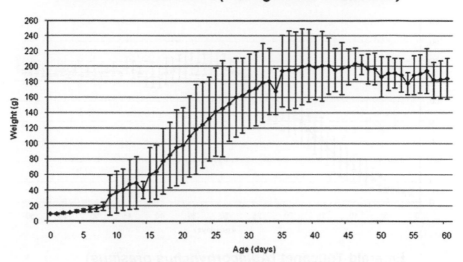

Saffron Toucanet (*Baillonius bailloni*)

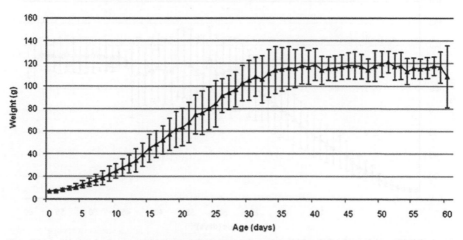

Fig. 5. Mean growth data for hand-fed chestnut-eared aracaris (mean ± SEM; n = 5, facilities = 2) and saffron toucanets (mean ± SEM; n = 24, facilities = 2) over the first 60 days of life.

a species weight chart.[5] As data from hand rearing of toucans expand, these growth curves can and should be enhanced to reduce band width and better evaluate variations in hand-rearing techniques.

Five of the 8 species had data from 2 facilities used in curve development. The keel bill toucan, collared aracari, and emerald toucanets were representative of the results of a single facility. None of the species selected were raised by all 3 facilities. Although absolute weight values varied, the shape of the growth curves was surprisingly similar for all species examined. Likewise, standard deviations did not expand when data from 2 facilities versus 1 were used for the construction of the growth curve.

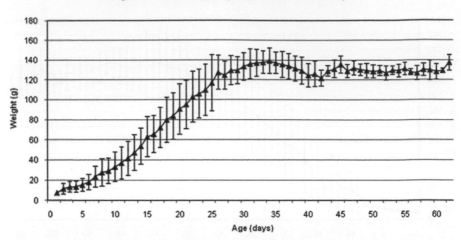

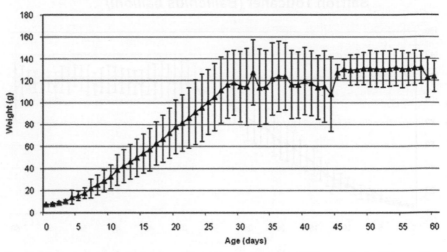

Fig. 6. Mean growth data for hand-fed Guyana (mean ± SEM; n = 8, facilities = 2) and emerald (mean ± SEM; n = 35, facilities = 1) toucanets over the first 60 days of life.

The limited number of birds used to produce the chestnut-eared aracari growth curve resulted in the largest percent standard deviation from the mean value curve. This limits the overall value of this curve as a comparison for any individual. It is hoped that as more of this species are produced and hand reared that a more focused curve can be produced.

The growth curves are all similar to previous curves produced for psittacine species based on growth data from 1 large facility.[4] The plateau phase approximates fledging with a later onset in the larger species. All weights from the plateau phase are lower than those published for free-living birds of the respective species.[1] It is likely that these are due to juvenile versus adult weights. There was a dip in weight for toco toucans around 50 days of age. Weight decreases at the time of fledging in other species may have been masked by the standard deviation or may not have occurred. Many of the species have dips in the mean weight around 42 days. These changes may indicate the time of tranistition. The time of transition to solid food can be associated with weight loss and birds should be watched closely to assure that illness is not involved.

Variability of incubation methods (all nest, nest/incubator, or all incubator) was not evaluated as it related to hatching success, chick size, or growth rates. Changes in incubation temperatures and humidity can impact success dramatically.[6] Further evaluations in incubation parameters with detailed notes will likely improve incubation techniques and hatching rates for these species. Likewise, parent-reared chicks were not compared to hand-reared chicks respective to growth. It is known that in psittacines, parent reared chicks are generally larger than their hand reared cohorts until the time of weaning. At weaning, the 2 systems of chick rearing become equivalent.[5]

Administration of nystatin is common to both RBZ and EFBG. While it is not documented in this study, it is a well-accepted part of hand feeding for toucans in most programs. Overgrowth of oral, proventricular, and ventricular *Candida* is a common concern in toucans. Management with Nystatin administration is effective but improvements in the protocols are possible. As with all facets of toucan hand rearing, an objective evaluation may be helpful.

Poor weight gains are a concern in all hand-rearing systems. Possible causes include insufficient feeding (formula insufficiently concentrated, or feedings too small or infrequent), dehydration, especially if chicks have recently suffered parental neglect, insufficient brooder temperatures, or illness.[7] Chick evaluations should include a review of the situation and the chick itself in addition to comparing the chick's weight against the growth curves. These curves are a tool in chick monitoring. It is hoped that the basics of rhamphastid handrearing presented here are a sufficient foundation to improve toucan husbandry and rearing.

ACKNOWLEDGMENTS

The authors thank Robert Seibels at Riverbanks Zoo and Jan Raines at Dallas World Aquarium for sharing the data that made this study possible. The authors also thank Julie Remp for original data management.

REFERENCES

1. Short L, Home J. Toucans, barbets, and honeyguides. Oxford (UK): Oxford University Press; 2001.
2. AZA Toucan Husbandry Manual. Available at: http://www.nashvillezoo.org/piciformes/toucan_husbandry.htm. Accessed March 2, 2012.
3. Groffen H, Watson R, Hammer S, et al. Analysis of growth rate variables and postfeeding regurgitation in hand-reared Spix's macaw (*Cyanopsitta spixii*) chicks. J Avian Med Surg 2008;22:189–98.
4. Clubb K, Skidmore D, Schubot R, et al. Growth rates of handfed psittacine chicks. In: Schubot R, Clubb K, Clubb S, editors. Psittacine aviculture: perspectives, techniques and research. Loxahatchee (FL): Aviculture Breeding and Research Center; 1992. p. 14-1–19.
5. Wolf P, Kamphues J. Hand rearing of pet birds: feeds, techniques and recommendations. J Anim Physiol Anim Nutr 2003;87:122–8.
6. Kuehler C, Kuhn M, McIlraith B, et al. Artificial incubation and hand-rearing of 'Alala (*Corvus hawaiiensis*) eggs removed from the wild. Zoo Biol 1994;13:257–66.
7. Vince M. Toucans. In: Gage L, Duerr R, editors. Hand-rearing birds. Ames (IA): Blackwell; 2007. p. 355–60.

General Principles of Nutrition for the Newly Hatched Chick

Elizabeth A. Koutsos, PhD

KEYWORDS

• Nutrition • Chick • Avian husbandry • Hydration • Diet

Feeding and care of a newly hatched chick require attention to a number of critical husbandry and management parameters, in addition to providing the appropriate nutrients in the appropriate form. There are a number of excellent resources related to these topics, notably, *Hand-Rearing Birds*.[1] This review will focus on the nutrient needs of avian neonates, although the aforementioned reference should be examined for species-specific details.

PRECOCIAL/ALTRICIAL SPECTRUM AND GASTROINTESTINAL TRACT DEVELOPMENT

Chicks hatch in a variety of stages of development, ranging from precocial, that is hatched with contour feathers, open eyes, able to leave the nest site and requiring no parental care, to altricial, or hatched with no plumage, closed eyes, and requiring parental investment in feeding and thermoregulation. There are numerous variations of these two extremes, and each variation represents an animal in a different stage of development.[2] Thus, it is likely that these chicks have different nutrient requirements to develop to a similar phase of life (eg, ready to fledge).

The timing of gastrointestinal tract development and onset of digestive capacity likely reflect differences in feeding strategy and pathogen load to which that species evolved.[3] Regardless of developmental stage at hatch, the chick must begin to process and utilize dietary inputs very quickly. In the precocial chicken, by 24 hours post-hatch, enterocytes have gained polarity and developed a brush border, while crypt invagination of the small intestine is complete by 48 hours post-hatch, and by 5 days post-hatch the villus cell number and surface area plateau.[4] In the altricial chick, the GI tract develops at a faster daily rate based on percentage body mass, compared to precocial chicks.[5,6] This observation may be related to the fact the earlier stage of development of the altricial chick at hatch (and thus more rapid development is needed to allow for nutrient uptake), or that precocial chicks divert

The author has nothing to disclose.

Mazuri Exotic Animal Nutrition, PMI Nutrition International, LLC, 100 Danforth Drive, Gray Summit, MO 63039, USA

E-mail address: Liz.koutsos@mazuri.com

more ingested energy toward locomotion, whereas altricial chicks do not have this requirement immediately post-hatch.

The capacity to digest and absorb nutrients from the GI tract also develops rapidly. In precocial chickens, by 72 to 96 hours post-hatch, digestive function and enzyme expression of enterocytes are functional,[4] although it may take longer for specific enzyme function to be optimized. Similarly, digestive efficiency increases rapidly with age in the altricial bird.[7,8] For example, in house sparrows, 15% of an oral glucose challenge was absorbed by 3 to 6 days post-hatch, while 30% was absorbed at 12 days post-hatch and 60% was absorbed in adult birds.[7] Enzyme activity is also responsive to dietary nutrient profile in altricial birds. House sparrows fed diets containing starch had higher starch-digesting enzyme activity than did birds fed starch-free diets.[9]

Fasting or delayed access to nutrition in the very early period post-hatch dramatically influences development of the GI tract in the precocial chicken.[10] A substantial body of literature has documented that access to nutrients via ingestion is critical for induction of digestive activity, bacterial colonization, development of a competent immune system, and yolk sac nutrient utilization (see review[11]). For example, in chicks that are fed immediately post-hatch, yolk lipids are transported to the small intestine and utilized at a much greater rate than if chicks have delayed access to feed, which results in greater transfer of yolk lipids directly into systemic circulation, thus bypassing the GI tract and reducing its rate of development.[12] Additionally, fasting or delayed access to diet-derived nutrients tends to favor colonization of the GI tract by pathogenic coliform bacteria.[13] Little work has been conducted on the effect of delayed access to feed in altricial chicks early post-hatch, although it is clear that like precocial chicks, altricial chicks hatch with yolk sac stores that are used during the first 24 to 48 hours post-hatch,[14] although yolk sacs may be of lower mass in the altricial chick than in the precocial chick.[15] Once the yolk sac is resorbed, the altricial chick appears to be very capable of handling periods of food restriction without concomitant reductions in the rate of GI tract development[16] and may result in enhanced small intestine surface area.[16]

There are clear differences in the stage of development for chicks that hatch along the precocial-altricial continuum. At the extremes, precocial chicks hatch with a GI tract that develops in size and function very rapidly in the days post-hatch. Altricial chicks hatch with relatively more developed GI tracts in proportion to the development of other tissues but also undergo a period of rapid growth and digestive capacity development. Precocial chicks have better utilization of yolk sac reserves and initiation of GI tract development when exposed to food early post-hatch, and this issue remains to be addressed in altricial chicks.

ESSENTIAL NUTRIENTS FOR CHICKS

An excellent review of avian nutrition is recommended for further reading in this area.[17] As in other taxa, birds require water, amino acids, fatty acids, vitamins, and minerals for growth and development. Moisture is critical to hatchling success, and moisture requirements are highest in the newly hatched chick and reduce over time, based on work on hand-reared cockatiels.[18] Similarly, in wild scarlet macaw chicks, moisture content of crop contents decreased significantly with increasing age.[19] A well-hydrated chick is evident by plumpness of skin, as opposed to a dehydrated chick in which the skin is generally tight, dull and dry **(Fig. 1)**.

After water, there is considerable debate as to the proper nutrient profile and form required by any given avian species. Most empirical studies have been conducted in precocial, granivorous domesticated poultry species including chickens, turkeys, and

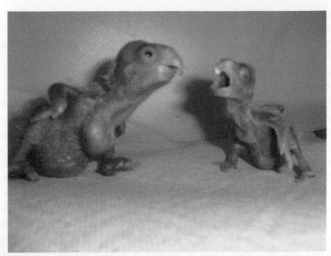

Fig. 1. Hydration and crop fill on chicks fed 2 handfeeding diets. The chick on the *left* is well hydrated and has a full crop, while the chick on the *right* is dehydrated and begging. Note the plump and shiny skin around the joints and the toes on the well-hydrated chick versus the drawn, wrinkled, and dull skin on the dehydrated chick.

quail.[20] Clearly, these species do not represent the diversity of development at hatch, nor the wild-type feeding strategies with which other species of birds have evolved. However, many of the empirically determined nutrient requirements can provide a reference by which species-specific differences can be based. For example, the protein and amino acid requirements for growth are based on the needs for protein accretion or synthesis of other metabolites, the rate of endogenous losses of proteins and amino acids, and the rate of oxidation and loss of nitrogen to other metabolic pathways.[17] These processes are likely similar across avian species for the first requirement (ie, needs for protein accretion) but different for the latter requirements (ie, rate of endogenous losses and oxidative/metabolic losses). Frugivorous and herbivorous birds tend to have lower rates of obligatory losses compared to granivores, while faunivores and carnivores tend to have higher rates of obligatory losses. Thus, the requirements for amino acids and nitrogen for growth may be similar, but the frugivore and herbivore may have lower overall protein requirements, while the faunivore may have higher overall protein requirements.[17] In all species, protein restrictions during growth are noticeable due to the essentiality of protein for feather and muscle production and result in lower growth rates and feather production in cases of deficiency or imbalance.

Lipids generally serve as an energy substrate and a source of essential fatty acids. For chicks with substantial flight requirements after fledging, lipids will be stored as future energy reserves, and the diet during development must provide the necessary precursors to meet these needs. The essential fatty acid requirements of most species of birds have not been determined. Chickens require linoleic acid,[20] and while most other avian species likely have the same or similar requirement, other fatty acids are probably essential as well. For example, birds that have evolved to eat fish and krill have adipose tissue that reflects a diet high in long chain omega-3 polyunsaturated fatty acids (PUFAs) and probably require a source of these PUFA in their diet.[17] Additionally, there is evidence that omega-3 PUFA may promote more optimal health status in granivorous birds,[21] and as such, feeding of omega-3 PUFA may be desirable in many avian species. More work is needed to fully characterize the optimal levels and types of fatty acids that promote optimal growth, health, and longevity in a variety of avian species.

Vitamins and minerals are required by all avian species, although the exact dietary concentration required has not been clarified for every avian species. However, poultry requirements can serve as a baseline by which levels can be set, and then species-specific knowledge may be applied to further refine these values. For example, sensitivity to iron in some species such as toucans[22] may necessitate the feeding of iron-controlled handfeeding formulations, although the requirement for iron in a developing chick is presumably much higher than that of an adult, and thus care must be taken to not underfeed this essential nutrient. In addition to general vitamin and mineral requirements, zinc and vitamin A and B_{12} levels directly affect intestinal development and deficiency or toxicity of these nutrients will impact the chick's ability to process other dietary components (see review[11]). Finally, calcium is essential for bone formation and, in flighted birds, may be the limiting factor for successful fledging and associated flight, food acquisition, and predator avoidance.[23] Bone length (and linear bone growth) influences the fledging time of chicks,[24] and these chicks also appear to preferentially calcify certain bones during development. The house wren was shown to preferentially calcify coracoid bones and leg bones, with lower calcification of wing bones, presumably to provide skeletal integrity for those bones that would receive the highest impacts during the fledging process.[23] Calcium is a primary concern in insect-eating chicks, since commercially available insects are generally deficient or imbalanced in calcium or calcium:phosphorus ratio, respectively.[25]

DIET STRATEGY AND GENERAL PRINCIPLES OF FEEDING CHICKS

Chicks may be raised by their parents, in which case parental diet inputs must meet the needs of the chicks, or they may be hand-raised. Hand-rearing of chicks may take place due to necessity (eg, rehab or fostered chicks) or by choice (eg, to encourage double clutching of certain species or for socialization of future pets). Psittacine chicks that were gently handled on a daily basis had lower stress responses to handling, and some changes in immune responses indicating lower overall stress levels.[26]

Many avian species provision their chicks with dietary components that differ from their typical adult diet items. This is due to several factors including higher nutrient requirements for the developing chick that cannot be satisfied by some adult-type diet items (eg, nectar and fruit may be limiting in protein/amino acids for growth and feather development), a need for physical processing of adult-type diet items that cannot be achieved by the neonatal chick due to an immature GI tract (eg, grinding of seeds may not be feasible with an immature gizzard[27]), limited ability to digest adult-type food items due to immature digestive enzyme functions (eg, starch-digesting enzymes may take time to be functional in the GI tract of the chicks), or limitations in excretory ability (eg, high salt marine food items fed to young chicks with limited capacity to divert energy for salt excretion).

FAUNIVORES

Faunivores feed on animal matter, and within this category are insectivores, plankto-nivores (eg, flamingos), piscivores, and carnivores.

Insectivores

Insectivorous birds consume a variety of insects, and this category includes obligate insectivores such as woodpeckers and some swallows, but also includes a number of frugivorous, nectarivorous, and granivorous birds that consume insects during the breeding season. For example, many passerine chicks are insectivorous during development and generally have insectivorous/granivorous or frugivorous diets as adults.[1]

It is difficult to generalize about the nutrient composition of insects, given their high variability due to the species and life stage of the insect. However, in general, insects are relatively high in crude protein (40%–70% dry matter basis [DMB]), although this value may include nonprotein nitrogen as in the case of insects with chitin exoskeletons.[28] Chitin may be digested by birds that have chitinase activity; this enzyme has been identified in common starlings, raptors, and some seabirds but is absent or low in chickens, psittacines, and pigeons.[17]

The fat content of insects is highly variable, ranging from 4% to 55% DMB,[28] and depends on the life stage and species of the insect in question. In general, larval insects contain much higher fat content than do adult insects (eg, mealworm larvae ~32.8% fat, DMB vs mealworm beetle ~18.4% fat, DMB[28]).

The calcium (Ca) content of insects is generally below the required level for adult or growing birds, while phosphorus (P) is often adequate, thus creating an imbalance of Ca:P. Gut loading of insects, the practice of feeding the insects a diet that will "fill" their GI tract and alter total nutrient content to provide balanced Ca:P has proved to be the most effective way to affect calcium levels in insects.[25] However, the level of calcium achieved in commercially available insects by gut loading may not be adequate for growth requirements, for which a 2:1 ratio of Ca:P may be optimal.[1] Calcium carbonate may be needed to be supplemented in the hand-rearing diet in these instances.

Given the large number of passerine chicks that are insectivorous during the nestling phase and are routinely hand-raised in rehabilitation settings, handfeeding diets have been developed to support their growth. The formula for nestling songbirds[29] has been tested and shown to support development of a number of avian species.[30]

Carnivores

Carnivores specifically feed on terrestrial vertebrates and generally provide their chicks with similar food items. Hand-rearing these animals generally involves feeding commercially available prey items including rodents.[1] The nutrient content of the prey items varies due to genetics, age, life stage, and sex of the prey animal. A comparison of nutrient composition of some prey items and the recommended nutrient intake for slow growing chickens demonstrates that prey items may contain lower nutrient levels than desired to meet the needs of growing animals (**Table 1**). However, some nutrients are reported to be able to be modified in the prey item in response to changing the dietary nutrient level.[31] For example, the lipid content of quail and rats was increased by feeding those animals higher dietary lipid levels.[32] Similarly, in rats, as dietary vitamin E level increased, so did tissue vitamin E level.[33] Increasing prey vitamin E content may be advantageous for the nutrition of the animals being fed. For example, Gyr-saker falcon hybrids fed 1-day-old chicks had higher plasma α-tocopherol than did birds fed turkey breast meat and reflects the fact that the 1-day-old chicks had higher vitamin E content (~400 IU/kg) than did the turkey breast meat (7.5 IU/kg).[34]

Table 1
Average composition of selected prey items compared to recommendations for slow-growing egg-type chickens

	Quail	Rats	Mice	Capelin	Atlantic Herring	Shrimp	NRC Slow Growing Egg-Type Chickens Adjusted for Caloric Density (kcal)			
	Mean	Mean	Mean	Mean	Mean	Mean	2900	4500	5500	6000
Moisture (%)	65	65	67	81	75	79	–	–	–	–
Lipid (%)	32	38	23	30	27	3	–	–	–	–
Protein (%)	72	66	63	66	57	77	17	26	32	35
Ash (%)	10	7	10	11	10	12	–	–	–	–
Vitamin A (IU/kg)	70,294	76,812	945,544	99,366	21,284	**286**	1500	2328	2845	3103
Vitamin E (IU/kg)	67	140	73	192	77	335	10	16	19	21
Ca (%)	3.4	2.7	3.6	1.7	**1.7**	2.6	0.9	1.4	1.7	1.9
Cu (mg/kg)	**2.6**	**1.6**	4.2	**6.5**	**5.0**	99.0	4.0	6.2	7.6	8.3
Mg (mg/kg)	**549**	**328**	**492**	1600	2900	2500	600	621	759	828
Fe (mg/kg)	75	47	101	88	98	188	60	93	114	124
Mn (mg/kg)	**6**	**2**	**5**	4	**5**	32	30	47	57	62
Zn (mg/kg)	**53**	30	**54**	**64**	62	77	35	54	66	72
Calculated kcal/kg	5734	6063	4743	5430	5929	4704	–	–	–	–

NRC recommendations are for chicks fed 2900 kcal/kg; calculated nutrient levels for higher caloric density diets are also shown. Data in bold represent values below the recommendations at an equivalent caloric basis. All data, except Moisture, are presented on a DMB.

Data from Refs.[20,32]; and Bernard JB, Allen ME. Feeding captive piscivorous animals: nutritional aspects of fish as food. Nutrition Advisory Group Handbook. Fact Sheet 005; 1997. Available at: http://www.nagonline.net/Technical%20Papers/NAGFS00597Fish-JONIFEB24,2002MODIFIED.pdf.

Piscivores

Piscivores consume diets composed of fish, and examples include pelicans, many storks, cormorants, mergansers, and osprey. These chicks should be provisioned with high protein animal matter including insects, fish, and rodents.[1] In the wild, some species that normally specialize on marine fish modify diets for their chicks to include more freshwater and terrestrial based diet items (eg, laughing gulls).[35] This is hypothesized to be related to salt intake; that is, due to the high energetic cost of salt excretion, minimizing salt intake of hatchlings allows energetic inputs to be directed toward growth[35] and warrants further investigation in hand-reared piscivorous chicks.

As with other food items, feeder fish are nutritionally very diverse. Species, life stage, age, sex, season, and the normal aquatic environment of the fish species in question have dramatic impacts on the nutritional composition (see, **Table 1**). For example, salmon harvested prior to completion of spawning have much higher lipid and caloric content than do fish harvested post-spawning, which will dramatically affect energy content and food intake levels.[36] Fatty acid profiles also vary dramatically between fish species and reflect environmental temperature and pressure,[37] food source, and age or size.[38] Thus, choosing the appropriate feeder fish for a particular chick requires thought as to its dietary requirements (eg, appropriate dietary n3:n6 fatty acid composition), as well as considerable laboratory analysis to account for the inherent variation in feeder fish nutrient composition.

FLORIVORES

Florivores consume plant matter and may be generalists or specialize in grasses (graminivore), grains and seeds (granivore), fruits (frugivore), and nectar (nectarivores), among others.

Granivores

Granivorous birds consume grains and hard seeds and include sparrows, finches, waxbills, some ducks, pigeons, and parrots.[17] Within the parrot family, most species consume some seeds, and some are exclusively granivorous including budgies, cockatiels, hyacinth macaw, red-fronted macaw, and black cockatoo. However, seed-based diets are generally not appropriate for the growth of granivorous chicks. In zebra finch chicks, body mass, feather development, and immunocompetence were retarded, and mortality was higher in chicks fed only seeds compared to those fed seeds plus hard-boiled egg (a source of protein, essential fatty acids, and vitamins).[39] Commercial formulations generally provide more consistent and balanced nutrition; however, since seed-eating birds need to have adequate gizzard/ventriculus function to process their adult-type diet, it is important that hand-reared chicks be provided some sort of physical substrate in order to stimulate gizzard/ventriculus development. Increasing particle size of the handfeeding formulation or introducing small particles (eg, seeds or pellets) gradually is recommended. In the wild, the crop contents of scarlet macaw chicks were significantly larger in particle size than typical handfeeding diets.[19]

Commercial formulations for granivores do work well[1] and are available in different energy levels, based on variable fat content (eg, high energy formulations contain higher fat levels). The level of fat fed to a particular species is generally proportional to body mass. Larger birds tend to have higher lipid in their nestling diets, and smaller birds tend to need lower lipid levels in their handfeeding formulations. Feeding a diet too low in fat will result in poor growth rates; a diet too high in fat (or energy in general) can result in liver pathology.[40] Using body weight as a guideline can be problematic, however, as some species seem to have lower energy requirements during growth and are more susceptible to pathology related to overfeeding of dietary lipids. Cockatoos are commonly reported to have hepatic lipidosis, morbidity, and mortality in response to feeding high-fat handfeeding diets. Additionally, it is clear that in the wild a variety of nutrient profiles are fed to developing chicks. Scarlet macaw chicks were sampled for crop contents from 13 to 77 days post-hatch and ranged from 13.7% to 47.3% fat (mean 28.6; DMB) and 9.6% to −31% protein (mean 23.5, DMB) and these ranges did not differ due to chick age.[19]

Parental Inputs cannot be ignored and may be difficult to replicate with prepared feeds. For example, IgA is secreted into the "crop milk" of pigeons, thus presenting an opportunity for transfer of passive immunity from hen to chick[41] or to provide local immunity in the gut environment as the chick develops a functional GI tract.[42] In addition to the antibody secretion, the secreted cells of the crop lining are rich in protein and fat and likely contribute to the nutrition of the developing chick.[27]

Frugivores and Nectarivores

Many birds that are frugivorous in their adult feeding strategy provide insects or other animal matter to their chicks to support growth and development.[1] In captivity, feeding of these chicks often requires similar adjustments to nutrient intake. For example, red bird of paradise, a predominantly frugivorous bird, was hand-reared using pinkies and dog food for the first 17 days post-hatch, after which a diet for frugivorous birds was introduced.[43]

Lorikeets and hummingbirds consume nectar as a primary diet component in the wild, but this food source will not provide adequate nutrition for development of chicks. Fruit flies are commonly fed to hummingbird chicks,[1] whereas lorikeets are successfully reared using granivore-type formulations.[1]

SUMMARY

Nutrition of the newly hatched chick is complex and requires an understanding of the wild-type feeding strategy of the species, the known nutrient requirements of birds, and appropriate application to the species in question. Next, composition of available food items, appropriate physical form, volume and frequency of food items, and desired end results (eg, appropriate fledging weight, ability to successfully find prey items or be socialized for human interactions, etc) need to be considered to provide the highest chance of successful fledging. There are several excellent resources to help guide the practical aspects of rearing chicks (eg, Gage and Duerr[1]), in addition to nutritional resources to guide a better understanding of the fundamentals of avian nutrition (eg, Klasing[17]).

REFERENCES

1. Gage LJ, Duerr RS, editors. Hand-rearing birds. Ames (IA): Blackwell Publishing; 2007.
2. Starck JM, Ricklefs RE. Patterns of development: the altricial-precocial spectrum. In: Starck JM, Ricklefs RE, editors. Avian growth and development: evolution within the altricial-precocial spectrum. New York: Oxford University Press; 1998. p. 3–30.
3. Jamroz D, Wiliczkiewicz A, Orda J, et al. Aspects of development of digestive activity of intestine in young chickens, ducks and geese. J Anim Physiol Anim Nutr (Berl) 2002;86(11–12):353–66.
4. Geyra A, Uni Z, Sklan D. Enterocyte dynamics and mucosal development in the posthatch chick. Poult Sci 2001;80(6):776–82.
5. Konarzewski M, Lilja C, Kozlowski J, et al. On the optimal-growth of the alimentary-tract in avian postembryonic development. J Zool 1990;222:89–101.
6. Sedinger JS. Growth and development of Canada goose goslings. Condor 1986; 88(2):169–80.
7. Brzek P, Caviedes-Vidal E, Hoefer K, et al. Effect of age and diet on total and paracellular glucose absorption in nestling house sparrows. Physiol Biochem Zool 2010;83(3):501–11.
8. Caviedes-Vidal E, Afik D, del Rio CM, et al. Dietary modulation of intestinal enzymes of the house sparrow (Passer domesticus): testing an adaptive hypothesis. Comp Biochem Phys A 2000;125(1):11–24.
9. Brzek P, Kohl K, Caviedes-Vidal E, et al. Developmental adjustments of house sparrow (Passer domesticus) nestlings to diet composition. J Exp Biol 2009;212(9): 1284–93.
10. Uni Z, Ganot S, Sklan D. Posthatch development of mucosal function in the broiler small intestine. Poult Sci 1998;77(1):75–82.

11. Koutsos EA, Arias VJ. Intestinal ecology: interactions among the gastrointestinal tract, nutrition, and the microflora. J Appl Poult Res 2006;15(1):161–73.
12. Noy Y, Sklan D. Yolk and exogenous feed utilization in the posthatch chick. Poult Sci 2001;80(10):1490–5.
13. Acheson DW, Luccioli S. Microbial-gut interactions in health and disease. Mucosal immune responses. Best practice & research. Clin Gastroenterol 2004;18(2):387–404.
14. Bancroft GT. Nutrient content of eggs and the energetics of clutch formation in the boat-tailed grackle. Auk 1985;102(1):43–8.
15. Vleck CM, Vleck D, Hoyt DF. Patterns of metabolism and growth in avian embryos. Am Zool 1980;20(2):405–16.
16. Konarzewski M, Starck JM. Effects of food shortage and oversupply on energy utilization, histology, and function of the gut in nestling song thrushes (Turdus philomelos). Physiol Biochem Zool 2000;73(4):416–27.
17. Klasing KC. Comparative avian nutrition. New York: CAB International; 1998.
18. Roudybush TE, Grau CR. Food and water interrelations and the protein requirement for growth of an altricial bird, the cockatiel (Nymphicus hollandicus). J Nutr 1986;116:552–9.
19. Brightsmith DJ, McDonald D, Matsafuji D, et al. Nutritional content of the diets of free-living scarlet macaw chicks in southeastern Peru. J Avian Med Surg 2010;24(1):9–23.
20. NRC, editor. Nutrient requirements of poultry. 9th edition. Washington, DC: National Academies Press; 1994.
21. Heinze CR. Effect of dietary omega-3 fatty acids on blood lipid composition and the inflammatory response in the cockatiel, Nymphicus hollandicus. Davis (CA): Nutritional Biology, University of California, Davis; 2010.
22. Dierenfeld ES, Pini MT, Sheppard C. Hemosiderosis and dietary iron in birds. J Nutr 1994;124:2685S–6S.
23. Dutta C, Johnson LS, Larkin D, et al. Skeletal development at the time of fledging in house wrens. Condor 1998;100(3):568–3.
24. Carrier DR, Auriemma J. A developmental constraint on the fledging time of birds. Biol J Linnean Soc 1992;47(1):61–77.
25. Finke M. Gut loading to enhance the nutrient content of insects as food for reptiles: a mathematical approach. Zoo Biol 2003;22:147–62.
26. Collette JC, Millam JR, Klasing KC, et al. Neonatal handling of Amazon parrots alters the stress response and immune function. Appl Anim Behav Sci 2000;66(4):335–49.
27. MacLeod A, Perlman J. Cream of the crop: an improved handrearing diet for hatchling and nestling columbids. J Wildl Rehab 2002;25:12–7.
28. Bernard JB, Allen ME, Ullrey DE. Feeding captive insectivorous animals: nutritional aspects of insects as food. 1997. Available at: http://www.nagonline.net/Technical%20Papers/NAGFS00397Insects-JONIFEB24,2002MODIFIED.pdf. Accessed March 24, 2012.
29. Finke M, Winn D. Formula for nestling songbirds (FoNS): updates for 2006. J Wildl Rehab 2004;27:3–4.
30. Sheldon LD, Drake A. Case study: a split-brood comparison of formula for nestling songbirds (FosNS) versus three facility-specific diets. Wildl Rehab Bull 2008;26(2):20–5.
31. Clawson AJ, Garlich JD, Coffey MT, et al. Nutritional, physiological, genetic, sex, and age effects on fat-free dry matter composition of the body in avian, fish and mammalian species: a review. J Anim Sci 1991;69:3617–44.

32. Clum NJ, Fitzpatrick MP, Dierenfeld ES. Effects of diet on nutritional content of whole vertebrate prey. Zoo Biol 1996;15:525–37.
33. Bendich A, Gabriel E, Machlin L. Dietary vitamin E requirement for optimum immune responses in the rat. J Nutr 1986;116:675–81.
34. Schink B, Hafez HM, Lierz M. Alpha-tocopherol in captive falcons: reference values and dietary impact. J Avian Med Surg 2008;22(2):99–102.
35. Dosch JJ. Diet of nestling laughing gulls in southern New Jersey. Colonial Waterbirds 1997;20(2):273–81.
36. Jonsson N, Jonsson B, Hansen LP. Changes in proximate composition and estimates of energetic costs during upstream migration and spawning in Atlantic salmon Salmo salar. J Anim Ecol 1997;66:425–36.
37. Cossins AR, Macdonald AG. The adaptation of biological membranes to temperature and pressure: fish from the deep and cold. J Bioenerget Biomembr 1989;21:115–35.
38. Iverson SJ, Frost KJ, Lang SLC. Fat content and fatty acid composition of forage fish and invertebrates in Prince William Sound, Alaska: factors contributing to among and within species variability. Marine Ecol Prog Series 2002;241:161–81.
39. Birkhead TR, Fletcher F, Pellatt EJ. Nestling diet, secondary sexual traits and fitness in the zebra finch. P Roy Soc Lond B Bio 1999;266(1417):385–90.
40. Davies RR. Avian liver disease: etiology and pathogenesis. Semin Avian Exot Pet 2000;9:115–25.
41. Goudswaard J, Van der donk JA, Van der Gaag I, et al. Peculiar IgA transfer in the pigeon from mother to squab. Dev Comp Immunol 1979;3:307–19.
42. Engberg RA, Kaspers B, Schranner I, et al. Quantification of the immunoglobulin classes IgG and IgA in the young and adult pigeon (Columba livia). Avian Pathol 1992;20:409–20.
43. Worth W, Hutchins M, Sheppard C, et al. Hand-rearing, growth, and development of the red bird of paradise (Paradisaea rubra) at the New York Zoological Park. Zoo Biol 1991;10(1):17–33.

Are There Long-Term Effects of Production-Based Rearing on Pet Bird Behavior?

Michelle Curtis Velasco, DVM, Dipl. ABVP-Avian Practice

KEYWORDS

- Pet Birds • Rearing • Handfeeding • Behavior
- Psittacines • Parrots

INTRODUCTION

The pet industry has long been attuned to keeping a ready supply of animals for public purchase. In the years prior to 1970, the majority of larger psittacine birds available for sale to the public were imported animals that were caught as young adults or nestlings from nests. As concern for the effect of this type of trade on native populations became publicized and yet at the same time the demand for exotic birds in the pet industry continued to grow, many individuals and pet suppliers began to collect many of these imported species and to set up pairs in the hope that they could breed parrots and try to fill this need domestically. Some astute breeders noted that psittacines kept in large full flight aviaries did not always start breeding right away. Pairs moved into more confined, usually suspended, cages often produced more offspring. Early clutches were often ignored by pairs just beginning to reproduce and losses could be high. By removing eggs or nestlings early after hatching, pairs would often return to the nests and double and triple clutch in a single year. The harvested babies were then incubator raised and expediently fed via feeding tubes or syringes until they could be marketed directly to either the new pet owners or pet stores.

The premise that handfeeding these babies would make them more bonded to the new owner and result in a very tame, loving pet was promoted as a superior product. Many pet owners wanted to finish the handfeeding process themselves, thinking that this would result in a closer bond with their pet. Unfortunately, the transfer of an unweaned baby bird to an inexperienced owner to raise was frequently problematic. This system generally results in the production of larger numbers of offspring to the pet trade, but losses through the process were probably higher in terms of morbidity

The author has nothing to disclose.
Fleming Island Pet Clinic, 4711 Highway 17, Building D, Fleming Island, FL 32003, USA
E-mail address: sunvet@bellsouth.net

Vet Clin Exot Anim 15 (2012) 205–214
http://dx.doi.org/10.1016/j.cvex.2012.04.001

and mortality. Inexperienced owners often do not realize when a baby is developing problems, have poor feeding technique, and lack knowledge of proper husbandry. Ultimately, this may result in a poor experience, which results in unhappiness and one less pet owner as a client for the entire industry.

During the time of mass importation, the greatest threats to aviculture from a veterinary standpoint were infectious in nature. Large-scale aviaries set up elaborate hatcheries and nurseries and paid extremely close attention to biosecurity and hygiene to prevent the introduction of infectious disease. These nurseries were often well lit, with individuals strictly separated and monitored for growth and health. Feedings were specifically timed and efficient. Unfortunately, this setup is closely reminiscent of the images of Romanian orphanages, which, while successful in helping reduce the death of infants born to HIV-infected mothers who either died or abandoned them, also resulted in multitudes of behavioral abnormalities arising from a lack of physical contact early in life. The Bucharest Early Intervention Study starting in 2000 noted that not only did orphans raised institutionally versus in foster home show behavioral disease, they also had changes in their DNA (shortening of telomeres) that the researchers thought were linked to early childhood adversity. While unclear what this would mean for the children's long-term health, earlier studies indicated increased risk for cardiovascular disease and cancer and premature aging.[1]

In the next step of the process, well-meaning purchasers of baby psittacines would lavish attention on their new baby bird, expecting to be rewarded for their efforts with an intelligent, loving, well-adjusted avian pet. Unfortunately, as the increasing volumes of literature on avian behavior problems will attest, this plan has not been without a detrimental aspect. Studies indicate that the "behavior of altricial and social brain species—those whose young strongly rely on early social interactions and adult care—are strongly influenced by early developmental events. It is during this time that the brain is most plastic and receptive to environmental surroundings: what an infant perceives and receives effectively sculpts his/her developing neuroethology. The problems arise when there is a "mismatch" between what an individual expects ecologically and evolutionarily and what is experienced in the social and ecological context."[2(p387)]

Avian behavior problems, including many self-damaging issues, have become part of the daily workload of the avian veterinary practitioner (**Fig. 1**). Some of the earliest cases noted dealt with the tendency of certain species to pull out, damage, or destroy their own feathering, with the African grey parrot and various cockatoo species being highly represented. Unfortunately, treatment of the mature bird once the behaviors have been established is often unrewarding. By attempting to correct the early mismatch at the breeder and production level, possibly the incidence of behavioral problems in the well-bred pet bird can be lessened.

As in any industry, there will be those individuals whose only concern is the earning of a profit. Fortunately, in many aspects of the animal industry, there are also those who work at lower compensation just to be around the animals they love. These breeders began to work on providing a more natural early environment. Keeping clutches together longer when possible, using towels to mimic the reassuring feel of a parent wing on a nestling's back, gradual introduction to stimuli, and even allowing young fledglings the opportunity to experience flight prior to the first wing clipping are all tools that could be used to help prevent some of the confusion described here.[3,4]

There are significant differences in the sociobiology of the different large psittacine bird species commonly raised and kept as pets. It has been widely recognized that many domestically produced African grey parrots have actually been selectively bred

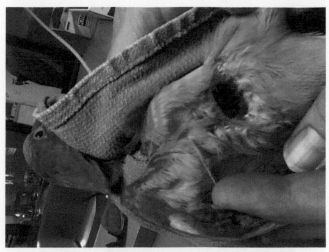

Fig. 1. Blue Quaker with self-mutilation injury. Previously hand fed, this is a very tame and loved pet.

to eventually exhibit feather destructive behavior. As with other pets such as dogs and cats, any issue that results in damage to the appearance of an animal results in owners seeking veterinary assistance often more quickly compared to other health problems. When a pet African grey began to damage its feathers, owners were often advised that the animal was sexually frustrated and should be set up for breeding. The well-adjusted, non–feather-plucking African grey was likely to stay in its happy home.

As patterns began to emerge in behavior, the link between highly cuddled handfed baby African greys and early-onset (9–18 months of age) feather destructive behavior (FDB) started to be recognized by astute avian practitioners. Young African greys that establish separation from petting contact (often by biting) appear less likely to start early FDB (Marge Wissman, DVM, NAVC, Orlando, FL, personal communication, January 1995). The author has also observed this in her practice. In addition to being less adapted to the pet home, some of these handfed African greys also had difficulty being productive in the breeding flock (**Fig. 2**).

To better understand how some of these early experiences may have long-lasting effects, we can look at some of the evolutionary strategies various species have developed to maximize reproductive success. The 2 general breeding strategies that animals tend to use are referred to as K-strategies and R-strategies. No 2 species exhibit exactly the same reproductive behavior but by examining the differences we can begin to elucidate some of the reasons for failure or success later in life for birds raised according to methods perhaps counter to their evolution. The theory hypothesizes that selection pressures work to drive species into evolving a strategy of producing many offspring with lower parental investment (R-strategists) or producing fewer offspring with greater parental investment in ensuring more individual offspring make it to adulthood (K-strategists). R-strategists rely on higher reproductive rates with less parental time investment and more instinctive survival skills. K-strategists tend to spend longer periods of time with their young and rely on intelligence and training of their young to increase survivability.

These species also tend to develop strong pair bonds and will often be more successful reproductively if allowed to self select their mate instead of being force

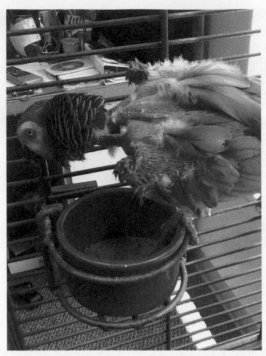

Fig. 2. A 20-year-old African grey parrot that was handfed by the owner and extremely bonded to him. This bird spends lots of time on the owner's shoulder and is frequently stroked on the back by the owner.

paired. Many of the larger psittacines such as macaws would be categorized as K-strategists. This would indicate that to have better, more successful breeders, we need to look back at their early experiences to maximize socialization and other life skills. While smaller psittacines, which would be more R-strategists, seem to be hard wired to survive, mate, and breed, the larger psittacines may seem to rely more on learning important behavior from their parents and other flock members.[5] It may be inferred then that chicks learn the skills to be a successful flock member from others around them and after weaning/fledging. For the pet bird, their flock consists of the owner and their household.

Observation of Moluccan cockatoos in nesting and rearing situations showed that parents were extremely attentive to newly hatched babies, feeding and grooming the nestlings as often as every 15 minutes. Both parents were rarely out of the nest for more than 15 minutes until fledging.[6] As the youngsters fledged, they were introduced to other similar-aged young birds in the flock and continued to learn social skills from peers as well as the immediate family group with competition for food and flighted play being major components of their physical and mental development.[7]

This differs greatly from the method used to raise many captive cockatoos. Hand-fed birds in a commercial aviary are quickly pushed to 2- or 3-times-daily feeding in sterile, sometimes well-lit incubators. Often this involves little physical contact outside of the actual feeding until they are transferred to the new owners at fledging or, even worse, sooner. These well-meaning owners lavish love and physical contact while doing very little to educate the young birds as to the rules and boundaries of living within the flock (now defined by the bird as its human family). Unfortunately, many instinctual behaviors then conflict with human flock expectations. Separation from the flock would necessitate calling and vocalization until reunited. This activity is interpreted as wanton screaming by the human flock, and rather than responding with reassurance, the young bird is sometimes ostracized or isolated in an attempt to control the behavior. Worse confusion can occur as sexual maturity arises and attempts are made by the cockatoo to bond to the affectionate human flock member chosen as a possible mate. Once again, the natural human response to this behavior is often not favorable and the young birds can truly become "sexually frustrated."

Unfortunately, the natural affectionate behavior of the umbrella cockatoo made them the obvious choice for pet owners whose needs included frequent touching and petting. These are behaviors that the normal Amazon parrot would not tolerate as it matured. Ironically, it is uncommon for Amazon parrots to present for purely behaviorally induced FDB. There have been many cases where hand-reared cockatoos or African greys that had no experience with other birds at fledging and reached sexual maturity in a pet situation are never able to adjust and breed successfully in an aviary situation.[5] They seem unable to recognize their mate as the same species as they have imprinted too strongly on humans. They may be unable to recognize and respond appropriately to interactions with other birds.

As avian medicine has continued to advance, nutrition and husbandry have improved dramatically. Preventative health care has become routine for birds, and increasingly available diagnostic testing and treatments have allowed earlier diagnosis and intervention. The most common chief complaints being presented to veterinarians in avian practice began to shift from the infectious disease issues to include behavioral disease problems. Avian veterinarians and other support individuals began to shift focus and attempt to address these trends. Avian behavior became a hot topic in literature, conferences, and Internet sources. Astute individuals started to experiment with behavior modification techniques. Some hospitals began to offer basic avian obedience training classes, and avian behavior consultants became available for in-home training, as well as Internet and telephone sessions. This is similar to what has happened in canine practice with a specialty board specifically for veterinary behaviorists now recognized by the American Veterinary Medical Association. Relinquishment or euthanasia due to behavior problems has increased greatly in that aspect as well. Studies have been done in dogs whereby early separation from the mother and litter was shown to increase undesirable behaviors such as destructiveness, excessive barking, fearfulness on walks, and possessiveness toward food and toys.[8]

Much public attention has been focused on the ills of mass production of purebred puppies for sale, and as a result most states passed laws forbidding the commercial sale of unweaned puppies. A few states have followed suit and established similar guidelines for bird sales. This is somewhat complicated by the fact that while most breeds of dogs mature at a similar rate and age, the many species of birds in the pet trade mature at different ages and have dramatically different social traits. Aviculture must address this issue or further regulation may be forthcoming. If simple husbandry methods during the fledging and juvenile stage of life can eliminate many of these behavioral problems from occurring, it would seem prudent to establish these as routine. Fortunately, some exotic bird breeders see the benefit of taking the needed steps to socialize young birds prior to introduction to a less-educated family. Unfortunately, this involves much more time and effort. It can be difficult to recoup the costs involved when competing with more mass production facilities.

Attempts to encourage this process by trying to add further regulation to pet animal producers is unlikely to help this problem. Public education to combat the handfeeding myth is one place to start. Another possibility would be the start of careful genetic selection to enhance behavioral traits to adapt certain large psittacine species to domestic life. A study on wild foxes in Russia showed that they could be domesticated in as little as 6 generations of selective breeding.[9] Marketing of a value-added product in the form of a well-adjusted youngster selectively bred for temperament and good health will depend on consumer education. No longer can aviculture just rely on any unwanted and unsuitable pet animals to provide the basis of breeding stock for pet production.

Some breeders and avian behaviorists have taken the initiative to research and develop handrearing protocols to improve the gap between evolutionary and ecological expectation and the actual experiences encountered in the early developmental phase. Guidelines for creating a happy and problem-free avian companion were laid out by Christine Davis.[10] Phoebe Linden[11] has written several articles in which she describes workable ways to raise young macaws to be less fearful and more curious, also developed physically by controlled flight. Linden stresses that there are 2 developmental prerequisites that must be met before successful fledging can occur. Birds must have the experiences as neonates of comfort, and as neophytes develop, visual skills lead to curiosity. Because stages of development are built on sequentially, if any experiences are missing, it may lead to problems later in life. Even in the preparatory phase prior to flight, many skills are developed, including athleticism, flight issues, and confidence. She emphasizes taking the process slowly as the bird indicates it is ready to progress. Her techniques include the use of graduated lighting, starting with very dim light and closed boxes and arranging for young birds to gradually explore their environment as their physical and visual skills develop. She strongly recommends gradual wing clipping to allow the experience of flight to develop confidence, problem solving, and athleticism.[11] Doolen states it is his opinion that much of the problem behavior he sees in practice results from imprinted birds not being allowed to fledge and develop strong flight skills. He also has found that some birds allowed to develop flight skills even later in life may reduce or resolve some of the problem behavior. Wing clipping is no longer performed in his practice[12] (**Fig. 3**).

When the importation of parrots was at its peak in the 1970s and 1980s, some importers and aviculturalists held back many of the less popular species and set up breeding pairs. The experience gained from raising common altricial species from eggs for sale as pets was applied to rarer, more difficult species. This resulted in successful preservation, even reintroduction, of some severely threatened species back into their native environment. In these cases, extreme care was taken to teach these parrots the behavioral tools to survive in a parrot flock or family and prevent them from imprinting on humans for the sake of future production.

Studies at University of California-Davis on co-parenting in orange winged Amazons may help guide breeders and aviculturalists toward researching setups whereby parent-raised birds are concurrently handled by humans very early in life and before fledging.[13] Individual breeder experiences with co-parenting Caiques have also been described.[14] After first learning about the early findings from the co-parenting studies, the author also experimented with a young pair of yellow Naped amazons that had bred and had eggs or young removed from the nest yearly for handfeeding and sale. By setting up a method to block the entrance to the nest by the parents when out foraging in the cage, she was able to interact with the young. Starting first by just

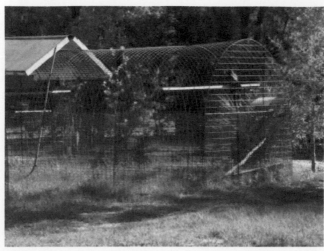

Fig. 3. Large flight cage for macaws can be used for breeding or exercising trained birds.

talking to the nestlings from outside the box, then later actually touching and handling the babies while allowing the parents to continue feeding them until almost normal fledging, the nestlings were afforded the opportunity to have both human and avian parents. Many of the young from this pair remained in the area and were seen by the author in her practice, and while not a scientific observation, it seemed that the parent-reared birds were just as tame and affectionate and better able to cope with stress and environmental change than those from the previous clutches.

In a study examining the effects of the rearing environment on the behavioral development of psittacines, 48 Nandays were raised in 4 different treatment groups. Groups included an enriched group that had chicks kept together in a colorful environment with soft toys and a view of the room. A restricted group was kept singly in tubs that were wrapped with brown paper. Handled groups were exposed to 15 minutes of gentle handling daily in addition to the routine feeding. Nonhandled birds had no additional handling other than routine feeding. Chicks' development was monitored through multiple parameters and then they were subjected to various tests including a novel object test, a novel conspecific test, an emergence test, an open field test, and a learning test. There was no evidence that the treatments affected their feather growth, final body weight, or age at weaning. However, both enrichment and handling significantly reduced the chicks' fear level in a variety of situations. Interestingly, the restricted nonhandled birds were less likely to approach a novel conspecific than any other group. The birds were then retested 4 weeks after weaning, which was about 16 weeks of age. This was after 9 weeks of infrequent handling. The handled birds were quicker to take a handheld treat and were more accepting of restraint. It was concluded this indicated a long-lasting effect of treatment. The researchers predict that enrichment and handling will improve the ability of a chick to adjust to captive life and reduce stress later in life.[15]

Veterinarians are able to educate owners of birds of any age concerning the use of enrichment at home. Learning is a never-ending process for birds that must adapt in the wild to ever-changing environments. Thus, providing enrichment throughout the bird's life, regardless of rearing technique, can only serve to improve their welfare and prevent or minimize behavioral issues. These enrichment techniques may start as

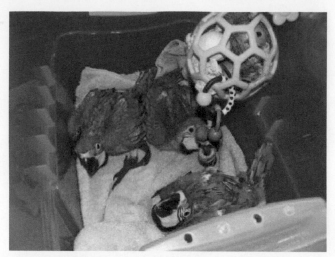

Fig. 4. Baby macaws raised together with toy for early enrichment.

early in life as possible and continue throughout adulthood. Various forms may afford the bird a choice in how it spends its time and interacts with others and its surroundings. Any activities or toys that provide a challenge can be included in an enrichment program, such as any methods of providing foraging opportunities, any socialization, and opportunities for bathing or grooming. The toys can range from simple to complex, limited only by an owner's imagination[16] (**Fig. 4**). Providing choice and solvable tasks such as through positive reinforcement training may help overcome some of the problem or negative behavioral issues seen in pet birds.[17]

As mentioned early, regulation regarding the sale of unweaned parrots is likely to have a negative effect by encouraging the practice of force weaning in order to expedite the weaning process. This entails prematurely reducing the frequency and volume of handfeeding formula with the belief that hunger will force the fledglings to eat on their own. This may predispose the fledglings to a multitude of behavioral problems including incessant begging in macaws and phobic behaviors in African grey parrots and possibly even contribute to cockatoo prolapse syndrome.[13]

Longer development times as well as expected longevity make the dangers of "puppy mill"–type production of large parrots even more disturbing as veterinarians, behaviorists, and loving caretakers take on the task of correcting behavioral problems that have their roots in very early experiences of the young bird. It is not the purpose of this article to condemn all producers of pet birds for practices that occurred in the past but rather to encourage them to pay attention not only to the physical needs of their product but also to their psychological and sociological needs as well. Pedigrees to identify behavioral trends that might make a certain line of birds better adapted socially to living within the boundaries of a human "flock" and then breeding to produce birds with those traits could be a consideration.

Veterinarians have a unique position to help guide breeders to select appropriate breeding stock and develop breeding programs geared toward production of a superior pet. Temperament is routinely mentioned in the selection of breeding stock for a variety of livestock, including horses, cattle, and domestic chickens. Aviculturists have certainly selectively bred for color and other feather mutations specifically to produce desirable pets. Smaller bird species such as cockatiels and lovebirds appear to have been unintentionally bred for egg production, resulting in health issues such as chronic egg laying and subsequent egg binding in the pet birds produced from this stock.

Public education regarding the dangers of improper early socialization might help justify the increased cost of appropriately raised animals. Education should also help improve husbandry to increase the quality of life for these birds throughout their lives. Addressing topics such as proper grooming techniques and activities such as foraging with owners of new birds ultimately results in better care and fewer problems later in life. Attending to the educational needs of highly intelligent, social creatures such as macaws and cockatoos should be as high on the priority for all those wishing to be involved in aviculture as nutrition, hygiene, and other, more obvious needs.[10]

REFERENCES

1. Rettner R. Harsh life of Romanian orphans damaged their DNA. Children's health. 2011. Available at: http://www.msnbc.msn.com/id/43061185/ns/health-childrens_health/t/harsh-life-romanian-orphans-damaged-their-dna/. Accessed April 17, 2012.
2. Bradshaw GA, Yenkowsky J, McCarthy E. Avian affective dysregulation: psychiatric models and treatment for parrots in captivity. Proceedings of the 30th conference of the Association of Avian Veterinarians. Milwaukee (WI). Bedford (TX): Association of Avian Veterinarians; 2009. p. 387–97.
3. Wilson L, Linden P, Lightfoot T. Concepts in behavior section, II: early psittacine behavior and development. In: Harrison G, Lightfoot T, editors. Clinical avian medicine, vol. 1. Palm Beach (FL): Spix Publishing; 2006. p. 60–72.
4. Linden PG. Fledging and flight for avian companions. In: Proceedings of the 20th conference of the AAV. New Orleans. Weatherford (TX): AAV Publications Office; 1999. p. 61–5.
5. Styles D. An overview of psittacine reproductive behavior and infertility problems. In: Proceedings of the 27th Conference of the AAV Avicultural Sessions. San Antonio (TX). Weatherford (TX): AAV Publications Office; 2006. p. 107–19.
6. Forshaw JM. Parrots of the world. New York: Doubleday & Company; 1973. p. 156.
7. Foster S. Behavioral anatomy of the male cockatoo. Parrothouse. Available at: http://www.parrothouse.com/sf10.html. Accessed April 17, 2012.
8. Pierantoni L, Albertini M, Pirrone F. Prevalence of owner-reported behaviors in dogs separated from the litter at two different ages. Vet Rec 2011;169:468.
9. Ratliff E. Taming the wild. National Geographic. 2011. Available at: http://ngm.nationalgeographic.com/2011/03/taming-wild-animals/ratliff-text. Accessed April 17, 2012.
10. Davis C. Creating a happy and problem-free avian companion. In: Proceedings of the 21st Conference of the Association of Avian Veterinarians. Portland (OR). Bedford (TX): Association of Avian Veterinarians; 2000. p. 43–7.
11. Linden PG. Teaching psittacine birds to learn. Semin Avian Exotic Pet Med 1999;8(4): 154–64.
12. Doolen M. A new perspective on fledging and wing clipping. In: Proceedings of the 27th Conference of the AAV. San Antonio (TX). Weatherford (TX): AAV Publications Office; 2006. p. 107–13.
13. Wilson L, Greene P, Lightfoot T. Concepts in behavior, II: early psittacine behavior and development. In: Clinical avian medicine, vol. 1. Palm Beach (FL): Spix Publishing; 2006. p. 60–72.
14. McMichael J. Co-parenting caique chicks. In: Bird talk. 2008. Available at: http://www.birdchannel.com/bird-magazines/bird-talk/2008-march/parenting-caique-chicks.aspx. Accessed April 17, 2012.

15. Luescher A, Sheehan K. Rearing environment and behavioral development of psittacine birds. In: Proceedings of the 25th conference of the AAV. New Orleans (LA). Weatherford (TX): AAV Publications Office; 2004. p. 297–8.
16. Joseph L. Enrichment for the avian patient. In: Proceedings of the 29th conference of the AAV. Savannah (GA). Weatherford (TX): AAV Publications Office; 2008. p. 123–9.
17. Joseph L. Empowerment and its importance in avian behavior. In: Proceedings of the 30th conference of the AAV. Milwaukee (WI). Weatherford (TX): AAV Publications Office; 2009. p. 403–6.

Cassowary Pediatrics

April Romagnano, PhD, DVM, DABVP (Avian Practice)[a,b,]*,
Richard Glenn Hood[c], Scott Snedeker, MD, DABIM[c],
Scott G. Martin, DVM, MS[b]

KEYWORDS
- Cassowary • Cassowary eggs • Avian veterinarian • Birds
- Pediatrics • Breeding

The cassowary is a keystone species on which the continued diversity of rainforest plants in Queensland, Australia, and nearby islands is vitally dependent. By latest estimates, fewer than 1500 birds remain in the Northern Region of Australia. Threats to cassowary survival around human habitation and in the wild include vehicles, dogs, feral pigs, habitat fragmentation and degradation, hunting, and natural disasters. Internal parasites (particularly ascarids), aspergillosis (*Aspergillus fumigatus*), and avian tuberculosis (*Mycobacterium avium*) are some of the infective agents that cull many immature birds (up to 12 months of age) in areas of compromised habitat. This has been seen in captivity as well.[1]

Our goal is to establish a more stable population of cassowaries, double and single wattle, than what we currently have in the United States. That population is tenuous at best but getting better. Our hope is to encourage others who have cassowaries in the United States to breed them successfully by raising these birds in an environment that more closely resembles their habitat for the general well-being of each individual bird. Perhaps in the future these captive bred birds may even be of value as a backup reservoir to Australia's population by providing new genetic diversity.

THERE ARE THREE SURVIVING SPECIES OF CASSOWARIES

The *Casuarius casuarius*, also known as the southern cassowary or double-wattled cassowary, is found in southern New Guinea, northeastern Australia, and the Aru Islands[2–5] (**Fig. 1**).

The authors have nothing to disclose.
[a] Avian & Exotic Clinic of Palm City, Inc, 4181 SW High Meadow Avenue, Palm City, FL 34990, USA
[b] Animal Health Clinic, Inc, 5500 Military Trail, Suite #40, Jupiter, FL 33458, USA
[c] The Cassowary Conservation Project, 3301 South Brocksmith Road, Fort Pierce, FL 34945, USA
* Corresponding author. Avian & Exotic Clinic of Palm City, Inc, 4181 SW High Meadow Avenue, Palm City, FL 34990.
E-mail address: drapril@scripps.edu

Vet Clin Exot Anim 15 (2012) 215–231
doi:10.1016/j.cvex.2012.02.002
1094-9194/12/$ – see front matter © 2012 Published by Elsevier Inc.

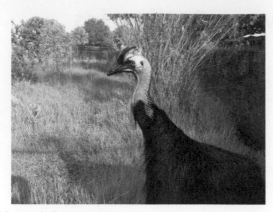

Fig. 1. Adult double-wattled cassowary.

The *Casuarius unappendiculatus,* also known as the northern cassowary or single-wattled cassowary, is found in northern and western New Guinea and in Yapen[2–5] (**Fig. 2**).

The *Casuarius bennetti*, also known as the dwarf cassowary or Bennett's cassowary (no wattle), is found in New Guinea, New Britain, and Yapen, mainly in highland[2–5] (**Fig. 3**).

NATURAL HABITAT

Cassowaries are native to the northern tropical rainforests of Australia, New Britain, Yapen, and Papua New Guinea. Single-wattled cassowaries are primarily from New Guinea and nearby smaller islands, while double-wattled cassowaries reside in the humid rainforests of northeastern Australia and New Guinea. Dwarf cassowaries are mainly found in the highlands in New Guinea, New Britain, and Yapen. Cassowary migration between New Guinea, New Britain, Yapen, northern Australia, and nearby smaller islands has been enhanced by centuries of trading by the indigenous human population[2–5] (**Figs. 4–6**).

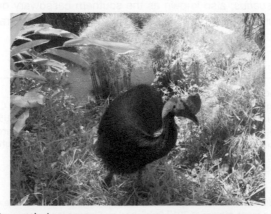

Fig. 2. Adult single-wattled cassowary.

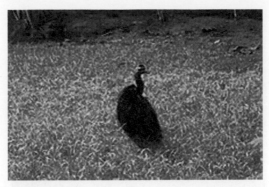

Fig. 3. Adult dwarf cassowary.

All 3 surviving subspecies of cassowaries are omnivorous but are predominantly frugivors. The natural diet of the cassowary comprises fruits, flowers, snails, and insects, as well as frogs, fish, mice, rats, carrion, and small birds.[2–5]

Cassowary chicks have been observed in the wild to eat the waste of adult male cassowaries.[5,6] Coprophagia may be a form of feeding from parent to young, hence an alternative strategy to regurgitation. This behavior has been observed in wild cockatoos, where neonates are fed their parents' feces. Ostrich chicks are also routinely observed consuming adult droppings. Coprophagia of adult male feces is not essential to cassowary chick viability, as captive chicks are typically raised from incubated eggs and have no access to either parent. Coprophagia, however, is practiced by captive raised cassowary chicks as well, which eat their own and their clutch mates' feces.

NONBREEDING/RESTING PERIOD

In the northern hemisphere, captive cassowaries rest from the beginning of August through mid-November. During this period, breeding adult birds are calmer and less

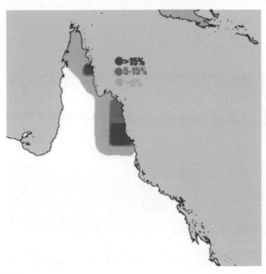

Fig. 4. Natural habitat.

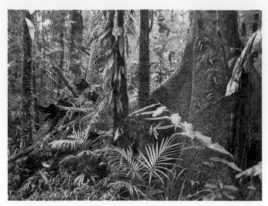

Fig. 5. Natural habitat rainforest.

interactive. Adult birds eat up to 5 gallons of peeled fruit and 4 cups of a protein source, such as dry pelleted dog food or monkey chow, each day.

Females and males of a breeding pair are best fed separately, as females may become aggressive while feeding. Females eat first and continue until they are sated. If fed together, males stand behind and to the side of the female while she eats. If a male gets between the female and food, she will hiss and kick him back into a submissive posture quite promptly and with apparent indignation. During this time, the males may occasionally take a few pieces of fruit.

As gravid female birds gorge, storing fat for egg development and production, the smaller males are typically deprived by their dominant hungry hens. Female cassowaries should be housed separately from their male mates during any periods of conflict. These periods vary and are dependent on the individuals. Careful observation of breeding pair behavior in this regard is key.

Cassowaries swim and relish frolicking in the water. They also mate in the water as well as on land.

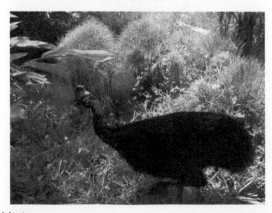

Fig. 6. Created habitat.

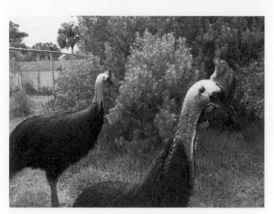

Fig. 7. Breeding pair.

PARENTAL HISTORY

It is important to keep records of the parents' diet, habitat, health, and breeding history. Note the condition of the parents' siblings if possible. Research for possible consanguinity between the breeding pair, as there are only a few bloodlines of cassowaries in the United States (R. Rundel, Denver Zoo and Natural Bridge Zoo, personal communication, December 2009). It would be ideal to obtain the history of offspring from previous seasons' clutches of the pair and any problems these chicks may have had during incubation, hatching, and maturation to help maximize future breeding success.

SEXUAL DIFFERENTIATION AND BREEDING

Cassowaries are predominantly sexually monomorphic. However, a few general characteristics help to determine a bird's sex. Generally, females are larger than males overall, especially in leg and foot proportion. At the beginning of the breeding season, female cassowaries are normally more aggressive than males (**Fig. 7**).

Since the first requirement for successful captive breeding is heterosexual or true pairs, gender determination is important for successful cassowary aviculture. The best options for sexing are blood DNA sexing for chicks and feather DNA sexing for adults.

Surgical sexing, the most accurate method of gender determination in monomorphic birds, is not recommended for cassowaries. Surgical sexing requires capture and anesthesia—a procedure that is not usually practical for adult cassowaries.

CLUTCHING: WILD VERSUS CAPTIVE

In the wild, the female cassowaries are polyandrous. They may have up to 4 different male mates serially in a single breeding season. The female lays approximately 16 eggs per breeding season. Each male cassowary, however, only breeds with a single female per breeding season.

After breeding, a female cassowary typically will lay up to 4 eggs per clutch in the nest prepared by the male. The male then drives off the female. The male subsequently dedicates the rest of the season to protecting, brooding, and hatching the eggs while the female seeks another mate. The male protects, feeds, and raises the young from the day they hatch to 14 to 16 months of age. Cassowary chicks are

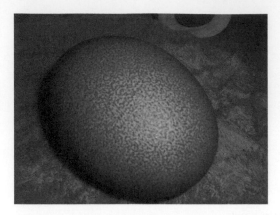

Fig. 8. Laid egg.

precocial and follow the father's lead—learning to forage for berries, fruit, small insects, amphibians, reptiles, rodents, carrion, and fish.

In captivity, a healthy female cassowary can lay up to 20 eggs if each egg is removed on the day it was laid. This equates to a 5-clutch breeding season in the wild. If each egg is removed promptly from a breeding pair, the female continues to mate with the male and he will continue to court her. Without eggs in his nest, the male will not begin brooding. Once the male begins brooding, either in captivity or the wild, he will become more aggressive and drive off the female. If the female is confined in captivity with the male when he is brooding, he may kill her.[2] However, the situation reverses if the female is finished with her ovulation and the male is still present in the same confined habitat. In this case she may attack and kill him.[2] Some pairs, however, can remain together peacefully in captivity year round. Caution and careful observation are prudent.

INCUBATION

In captivity, cassowary eggs should be collected on day 1. This improves clutch size for the season, and prevents predators, environmental conditions, or parental conflict from damaging the eggs.

Successful artificial incubation is dependent on several parameters once the eggs are taken from the parents. These include egg rotation, temperature, humidity, vibration, and airflow in the incubator. Once incubation starts, it must be continued within strict parameters and consistent environmental conditions[7,8] (**Fig. 8**).

EGG ROTATION

A Georgia Quail Farm Sportsman Model 1536 (GQF Manufacturing, Savannah, GA, USA) is a ratite incubator for ostriches and emus that has been found to be consistently effective for incubating cassowaries and is used by the authors. This incubator automatically turns the eggs alternately 180° every 3 hours on the egg's long axis. Good-quality incubators use timed mechanical turners with an average turn frequency of 10 hemirevolutions per day (**Fig. 9**).

INCUBATOR TEMPERATURE

Carefully maintaining temperature settings between 97.0°F and 97.5°F yields excellent chick viability. Historically, incubation temperature and humidity have varied for

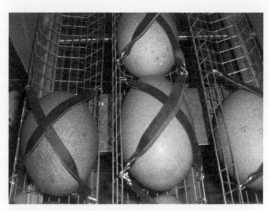

Fig. 9. Eggs in incubator.

different avian species, with settings ranging from 98.9°F to 99.3°F (37.3°C) with 30% to 45% humidity. It should be noted that viability of cassowary embryos using these parameters has been very poor (~3%). Considerably higher humidity settings (see later) and lower temperature settings have resulted in a much higher average embryo viability and chick hatching rate of 45%.

HUMIDITY

High cassowary chick viability is attributed to humidity settings being carefully monitored and kept between 57% and 64%. Any greater humidity fosters the development of "wet chicks." These chicks often drown at pipping due to excessive liquid albumin. Moreover, they are often edematous and as a result weak and slow to stand after hatching. Conversely, eggs exposed to low humidity may dry out, causing adherence of the shell membrane to the chick, preventing normal pipping. Incubator humidity is maintained by a reservoir within the incubator with capillary wicks supplied by a gravity siphon and a circulating fan. Wicks must be reversed daily to maintain a constant rate of evaporation. The ideal conditions in the incubation room should be maintained between 73°F to 75°F (22.5°C) and 43% to 48% humidity.

WEIGHT AND STRUCTURAL CHANGES DURING DEVELOPMENT

A healthy developing cassowary egg normally loses a small fraction of its water weight by diffusion during incubation (day 1 to external pip). Further data with regard to changes in egg weight during incubation are being collected. The air cell enlarges normally at the larger end of the egg between the inner and outer shell membrane as the egg loses weight during incubation. If the humidity is too high, the air cell will be small. If humidity is too low, the air cell will be larger. Rundel finds that 12% to 15% egg weight loss over incubation is most successful, but a range of 12% to 20% weight loss has resulted in live hatches.[7]

Washing of eggs, as is typically done in the poultry industry, could potentially reduce the viability of cassowary eggs.[9] The eggs are usually kept relatively clean in the nest by the male.

Artificially incubated eggs can be candled to monitor development. Due to the dark pigmentation and shell thickness, an extremely strong light source and a completely darkened room are required. An egg with a viable embryo at 3 weeks' development will have a clear shadow margin at the air space/liquid albumin compartments separated by the inner shell membrane (amnion). An infertile egg will have a hazy uneven shadow margin separating the air space/liquid albumin compartments with lucent streaks extending perpendicularly from the amnion in to the liquid albumin.

At 5 weeks, an infertile egg often will have a larger air cell than an egg containing a developing embryo. On rare occasions, an infertile egg will have a tiny air cell. Most artificially incubated live hatches have nearly exactly the same size air cell. An infertile egg will also cool faster during handling than a live egg after 5 weeks. Eggs are removed and observed daily after 6 weeks of incubation. Eggs are listened to, placed on a hard smooth surface to observe for movement, and checked for rate of cooling. By 65 days an egg may be removed from the incubator without prohibitive risk of discarding a viable embryo.

HATCHING

Hatching occurs between days 48 and 56. The egg will begin to have spontaneous movements, wiggling, spinning, or even hopping from 12 hours to as long as 14 days prior to hatching. This can be best observed by placing the egg on a smooth hard surface and closely monitoring it for 10 minutes.

Stages of Hatching

Just before hatching begins, a normal cassowary embryo assumes the hatching position with its head below the air cell close to the right wing tip. This is similar to other avian embryos. Internal pipping occurs toward the end of this stage.

It is assumed that a buildup of CO_2 causes the hatching muscle in the neck of the cassowary embryo to twitch. This is common to amniotes. This twitch causes the beak to penetrate the chorioallantoic membrane (ie, internal pip). At this point, the embryo becomes a chick—defined as such when it begins to breathe air within the air cell. A chirping sound may be heard from the egg as the lungs begin to function.[9]

Twitching of the abdominal muscles, which occurs secondary to breathing, causes the exteriorized yolk sac to be drawn into the chick's abdomen and cracking of the shell. This is the equivalent of external pipping, as cassowary chicks do not have an egg tooth with which to pip. With subsequent breaths, the level of CO_2 within the air cell rises. External "pipping" needs to happen soon to prevent death from suffocation.

Unlike psittacines, which are moved to a hatcher, cassowary eggs should remain in the incubator at 57% to 64% humidity. Humidity above 80% during hatching can result in edematous chicks that drown within the egg. Environmental parameters during hatching should not be altered from those during incubation as with other species. Additionally, at this time, turning of the egg should cease and it should be placed on the bottom of the incubator.

If the chick is unable to hatch within 1 to 2 hours, assistance should be provided. This procedure should be initiated only after a chick's chirping is heard within the air cell. To do so, identify the air cell by candling, and swab with 4% chlorhexidine solution and then open the center of the air cell with a sterile punch. Snip a small opening in the outer shell membrane with sterile surgical scissors and then very carefully break off bits of shell to open the air cell. Exercise care not to cause bleeding of the outer shell membrane (allantoic) and to avoid contaminating or injuring the chick with the instruments (**Fig. 10**).

Normally, the chick then emerges on its own unassisted. Most chicks chirp loudly while sitting on very large bellies filled with yolk. Often the yolk sac is too large for the chick to stand the first day or 2. Most chicks stand by day 2 as the yolk sac is absorbed. Nearly all chicks can stand by day 3. Some, however, walk early within

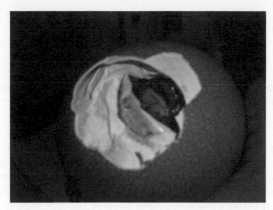

Fig. 10. Assisted hatching.

hours of hatching. In the wild, all chicks are up within hours of hatching. Posthatch activity does depend on clutch size as the male will not leave the nest until all chicks are hatched. In general, cassowary chicks in captivity may take 6 hours to 3 days to walk after hatching (**Fig. 11**).

Embryo and Chick Mortality

During early incubation, mortality may result from numerous factors, including failure of the parents and/or the artificial incubator.[9] Some common causes are improperly incubated eggs, inbreeding, genetic abnormalities, egg-borne infections, or contamination.

Additional causes of early embryonic death during artificial incubation include improper handling, excessive or insufficient temperature or humidity, excessive vibrations, improper egg turning, poor ventilation resulting in hypercapneic levels of CO_2, and malpositioning.[9]

Two of the most common malpositions are having the head aberrantly located at the small end of the egg or having the beak rotated away from the air cell. Eggs incubated below optimum temperatures develop more slowly and typically have

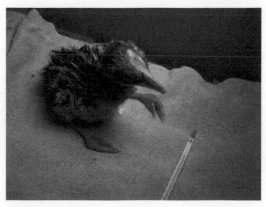

Fig. 11. Newly hatched chick.

increased problems with hatching. High or low humidity can result in the complications previously mentioned.[9]

All dead eggs should be necropsied. During the gross necropsy, the embryo's general condition and position are assessed. Abnormal tissues and fluids are cultured and/or sent off for histopathology. The shell is examined for color, texture, shape, and the presence or absence of stress lines. Thickness of the shell and degree of porosity are assessed by differences in texture.[9]

Hatchlings

Hatchling walking surfaces should be very soft and not slippery. Foam camping pads under towels are ideal. Heat lamps 18 inches above the floor keep the chicks warm. Chicks can lie under the light or move if they get too warm. Warm chicks lie down to sleep. Cold chicks cry and run around looking for warmth. A standard poultry waterer and small plate work well for watering and feeding.

Older siblings may reject younger nest mates. Eggs are laid 3 to 8 days apart. Hatchings are similarly spaced, so chicks will be of different ages. Chicks do imprint at this stage. A cassowary that imprints on a human may not breed with its own species and kill other members in the same enclosure. Care should be taken to minimize opportunity for chicks to imprint on keepers. In wild clutches, hatching is synchronized by delaying brooding and incubation until the last egg is laid.

The Pen

Incubator-hatched cassowary chicks should be kept in a climate-controlled space in captivity. The temperature should be maintained at 82°F (27°C) with 45% humidity. These spaces or pens should be fitted with appropriate footing as described earlier. Having the chicks on a surface that is too hard or slippery may cause injury to the hock or tibial-tarsal joint (**Fig. 12**).

Once the chicks reach 8 to 10 lb, they can be moved to a larger protected area fitted with rubber mats. After 1 year of age and a weight of about 40 lb, they can be moved to an outdoor habitat (**Fig. 13**).

Diet

Most chicks will not start eating until day 2 or 3, but some start on day 1. In the first 3 to 6 weeks, their appetites increase. The diet is predominantly composed of

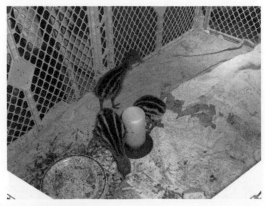

Fig. 12. Chicks in their padded playpen.

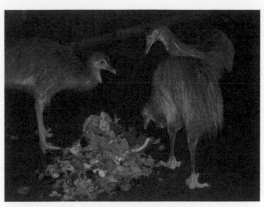

Fig. 13. Stable with rubber mats and 6-month-old chicks.

fruit (**Box 1**). A diet too high in protein may cause joint deformities (see Perosis). The chicks should finish their entire feeding in 30 minutes. After about the first 10 minutes of the meal, partially digested food passes from the cloaca as feces to be eaten again. In this way the food makes at least 4 to 6 passes through the entire digestive tract over 3 to 5 hours. After repeated processing, the waste loses its fruity color and appeal and is finally ignored. The authors speculate that this is a food gathering strategy in the wild as pet cassowaries in New Guinea households are observed to return in the same cache outside to excrete.

Coloring

Hatched chicks have gold and dark brown striped downy feathers covering the head and body. The legs and feet are pink. The casque spot is flat (**Fig. 15**).

By 12 weeks, the stripes fade to a solid golden brown, quite similar to the coloring of Sand hill crane chicks of the same age. The down disappears from the head from the top downward and the casque begins to dome (**Fig. 16**).

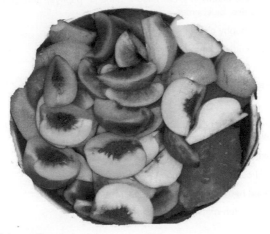

Fig. 14. Typical adult meal.

| Box 1 |
| Diet at different ages |

Days 1–3 hatching

- Typically do not eat or drink for 1–3 days

Days 4–7

- 3 tablespoons very small berries, minced fruit 5–10 mm in diameter daily
- Will scoop water with their beaks

Days 8–15

- 4 tablespoons very small berries, minced fruit including elderberries, raspberries, blueberries, blackberries, minced grapes, minced guava, minced banana, watermelon, cantaloupe, minced kiwifruit 5 to 10 mm in diameter daily
- 2–3 pellets of soaked puppy chow daily
- ¼ teaspoon shaved cuttlebone sprinkled on food daily
- Chicks will eat their clutch-mates' and their own feces.

Days 16–30

- 1 cup very small berries, minced fruit 5–10 mm in diameter daily
- 6 pellets of soaked puppy chow daily
- ¼ teaspoon shaved cuttlebone sprinkled on food daily
- ½ cup fine chopped baby greens daily
- Chicks will eat their clutch-mates' and their own feces.

Days 31–60

- 2–3 cups very small berries, minced fruit 8–15 mm in diameter daily
- 12 pellets of soaked puppy chow daily
- ½ teaspoon shaved cuttlebone sprinkled on food daily
- 1 cup fine chopped baby greens daily
- Chicks will eat their clutch-mates' and their own feces.

Days 60–90

- 2 cups halved grapes, cherries, 2-cm melon, banana, papaya, and guava chunks, whole raspberries, blackberries, blueberries
- 12 pellets of soaked puppy chow daily
- ½ teaspoon shaved cuttlebone sprinkled on food daily
- 1 cup fine chopped baby greens daily
- Chicks will eat their clutch-mates' and their own feces

Days 91–120

- 2½–3 cups halved grapes, cherries, 2-cm melon, banana, papaya, and guava chunks, whole raspberries, blackberries, blueberries
- 16 pellets of soaked puppy chow daily
- 1 teaspoon shaved cuttlebone sprinkled on food daily
- 2 cups fine chopped baby greens daily
- Chicks will eat their clutch-mates' and their own feces

121 Days to 6 months

- 4 cups whole grapes, cherries, strawberries, melon and papaya wedges for pecking, whole peeled banana and guava chunks, whole raspberries, blackberries, and blueberries
- 1 cup pellets of soaked puppy chow daily
- 1 teaspoon shaved cuttlebone sprinkled on food daily
- 3–4 cups whole baby greens daily
- Chicks will eat their clutch-mates' and their own feces

6–18 Months

- 2 gallons of any peeled fruit or berries (except avocado) in 5-cm pie
- 3 cups high protein dog food, fish food, or monkey chow daily
- 4–5 cups whole greens daily
- Chicks will eat their clutch-mates' and their own feces.

19 months to adults

- 5 gallons of peeled fruit, peeled melon halves, bananas. Nearly any produce is relished.
- 4 cups high protein dog food, fish food, or monkey chow daily
- All greens available
- Have not been observed to ingest gastroliths. We have not seen either adults or juveniles swallow foreign bodies.

Fig. 14 displays typical meal for an adult

By 12 months, the feathers will start to turn black and the skin of the head and wattles will start to acquire a blue and red color. The head and neck are nearly bald, and the casque becomes more prominent. The skin of the legs darkens to a charcoal gray (**Fig. 17**).

By 3 years, the cassowaries have deep vibrant adult coloring (glossy black feathers and iridescent blue, red, yellow, and orange coloring of the skin of the head, neck and wattle). The casque is now 3 to 5 inches tall.

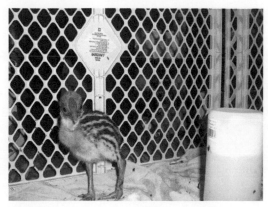

Fig. 15. One-week-old chick.

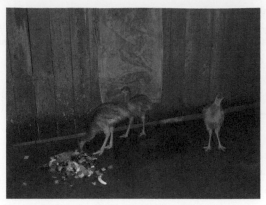

Fig. 16. Twelve-week-old chicks with golden breast feathers.

Physical Examination

Cassowary hatchlings are precocial. Physical examination of the chick entails assessing overall appearance, proportions, weight changes, gait, activity joint swelling, and social behavior. It is important to monitor for normal eating, defecating, color, consistency, and volume of its droppings and coprophagia.[8-11]

Remove abnormal chicks from the clutch early to prevent infection of the group and allow a more thorough evaluation. A chick that stops eating, becomes weak, is unable to stand, or inflates its neck air sacs (a distress display) may be demonstrating signs of an illness, injury or congenital malformation. A treatment plan may then be developed based on specific problems present. Delay of appropriate treatment may lead to mortality.[8-11]

Common Pediatric Problems

Unretracted yolk sac

Unretracted yolk sac has been seen most commonly in malpositioned chicks. Hatching may begin as soon as 12 hours and as late as 3 weeks after the first egg

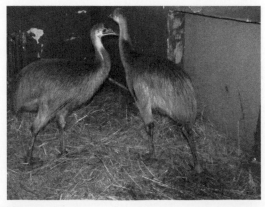

Fig. 17. Yearling chicks.

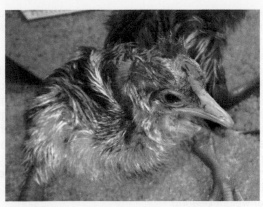

Fig. 18. Splay leg deformity.

movement is observed. Thus it is best to leave them unassisted until they are peeping in the air cell to avoid intervening prematurely. Premature intervention commonly results in an unretracted yolk sac and an underdeveloped chick. The yolk sac, a diverticulum of the small intestine, is normally internalized into the abdomen before hatching. The yolk sac is absorbed over the next few days, providing the chicks with nourishment and maternal antibodies. A prolonged retention of the yolk sac within the coelom can occur in cassowary chicks.[8–10]

Chicks with unretracted yolk sacs, and therefore an open umbilicus, should be placed on clean towels in the incubator and their umbilicus swabbed with chlorhexidine scrub. Crop and cloacal cultures should be taken, as well as yolk sac cultures if the latter is leaking. Chicks should be placed on appropriate antibiotics and oral antifungals. Chicks should also be treated with fluids. If the yolk sac fails to become internalized over 2 days, then surgery is necessary to amputate or remove the yolk sac.[8–10]

Splay leg deformities

Abduction at the stifle joint is a common deformity upon hatching often referred to as splay leg. One possible cause hypothesized is larger yolk sacs force apart the cassowary chick's legs (**Fig. 18**).

Splay leg is most common in the first 2 or 3 chicks of the season. Usually 1 leg is affected but both can be involved. Treatment is generally successful with bandaging techniques. This is done by hobbling with bandage tape (above the hock) for 3 days and observing closely for correct alignment.[8,9]

Perosis

Juveniles may also experience perosis or subluxation of the extensor tendon out of the tibial tarsal groove. Slippery or unpadded surfaces, trauma to the delicate joint capsule, and diets too high in protein and calories are suspect. The joint capsule, tendons, and articular surfaces are very delicate. Slipping and striking the tibial tarsal joint directly can cause rupture of the joint capsule. Direct injury to the extensor tendon can cause it to swell and result in subluxation, forcing it out of the tibial tarsal groove. Heel strike on a hard surface can cause the posterior articular tarsal groove to swell and thus cause the groove to "fill in," forcing out the extensor tendon. The tendon can be pushed laterally or medially. Clinical signs include hock swelling, limping, pronation, and inability of the chick to stand and extend the hock joint. A similar surgical procedure can be used for correction of either deformity.[5]

Some presubluxations with swollen joint capsules may respond to improved padded walking surfaces that allow more foot traction and absorb shock. Subtle subluxations also may respond to improved footing combined with physical therapy. This physical therapy also includes moving the birds to larger pens and encouraging increased walking and running activity. Exercise on safe walking surfaces is known to be of importance in such cases. Without external stimulation to move about, chicks that remained less or inactive would stop gaining weight and decline in health. While birds sustaining severe subluxations are typically euthanized, surgical correction of severe subluxations as a means of providing weight-bearing function is possible. This procedure has often proved effective reducing the need for euthanasia.

Perosis, also known as slipped tendon, results in a swollen hock creating a deformity of the medial tarsal and tarsal metatarsal bones. The tendon can luxate medially or laterally. Luxations can create joint deformities that render the limb incapable of normal weight bearing.

For surgical correction, a lateral paramedian incision is made through the skin over the caudolateral aspect of the joint midway between the lateral condyle of the tibiotarsus and the displaced tendon. The incision extends in a proximal and distal direction over the tibial tarsal joint to expose the displaced tendon. The tendon is dissected free from any trochlear and medial adhesions to the skin and subcutaneous tissues. Once the tendon is freed, make a lateral incision over the joint capsule to expose the tibial tarsal joint. Subsequently, dissect the tendon free of any additional medial attachments to alleviate tension that may pull the tendon from the trochlear groove. Begin this stage with freeing the tendon proximally from the tibial tarsal bone—similar to a quadriceps release. The trochlear groove should be examined and, if it is shallow, a block wedge resection can be performed easily with a scalpel blade to deepen the groove, which will assist in maintaining reduction. The tendon is then replaced to its normal position within the trochlear groove of the tibial tarsal joint. The tendon contains a sesamoid bone that resides in the trochlear groove of the tibial tarsal joint. The tendon is then secured in its normal position in the trochlear groove by suturing the tendon sheath to the lateral retinaculum of the joint capsule and periostium with 3-0 absorbable suture in a simple interrupted pattern. Last, close the skin in a single layer with an interrupted pattern using a 3-0 nonabsorbable suture. The leg is bandaged routinely and splinted using a tongue depressor. Change the bandage weekly for 2 to 3 weeks before final removal of the dressing.

Eye malformation
Unilateral micro-ophthalmia has been noted in cassowaries (n = 1). No other complications were associated. The affected chick was viable and grew to adult size.

REPRODUCTIVE DISEASES AND BEHAVIORS
Female

Infertility
Infertility of the female cassowary may be due to nutritional issues such as a diet deficient in fruit. Female cassowaries tend to become more aggressive and irritable a few hours before egg laying. Eggs are typically laid in the afternoon.

Egg binding and dystocia
Egg binding, the most common obstetric complication of birds, has been noted in captive cassowaries. Egg binding can lead to death in the untreated hen. The typical cassowary egg-laying interval is between 3 and 8 days.

Dystocia, the mechanical obstruction of an egg in the caudal reproductive tract, which can result in cloacal impaction and/or prolapse, has also been seen and corrected in captive cassowaries. The handlers at the Rundel collection in Sonoma manually replace a prolapsed cloaca using a manual reduction technique similar to that used by cattlemen for a prolapsed uterus in a cow. This technique was used to allow treatment without veterinary assistance.

Male

Infertility

Infertility of the male cassowary may be due to a nutritional issue such as a diet deficient in fruit. Males also can be intimidated by an aggressive domineering female cassowary and not copulate with her.

Inbreeding

Inbreeding has been observed to be associated with poor chick viability in captivity.

SUMMARY

Abduction at the stifle joint is a common deformity upon hatching often referred to as splay leg. One possible cause hypothesized is larger yolk sacs force apart the cassowary chick's legs (see **Fig. 17**). Splay leg is most common in the first 2 or 3 chicks of the season. Usually 1 leg is affected but both can be involved. Treatment is generally successful with bandaging techniques. This is done by hobbling with bandage tape. (above the hock) for 3 days and observing closely for correct alignment.[8,10]

REFERENCES

1. Ollssen A. The impact of disease on free living cassowary populations in far North Queensland. In: Proceedings of Wildlife Disease Association International Conference. Queensland (Australia): Boongarry Veterinary Services; 2005. p. 199.
2. Perron R. The cassowary in captivity. International Zoo News 1992;39/7:No. 240. Available at: http://www.species.net/Aves/Cassowary.html. Accessed October 28, 2011.
3. Mack A, Wright D. Cassowaries in the Papua New Guinea rainforests. Cassowary Summit Proceedings. 2009. Available at: http://www.wettropics.gov.au/wwc/wwc_pdfs/CRT/CSummitProceedingsFinal.pdf. Accessed February 15, 2012.
4. Speer B. Ratite medicine and surgery. In: Proceedings of the North American Veterinary Conference. Orlando, 2006. p. 1593–7.
5. Smith DA. Ratites: Tinamiformes (Tinamous) and Struthioniformes, Rheiiformes, Cassuariformes (ostriches, emus, cassowaries, and kiwis) In: Fowler ME, Miller RE, editors. Zoo and wild animal medicine. 5th edition. Philadelphia: WB Saunders; 1999. p. 94–102.
6. Romagnano A. Mate trauma. In: Leusher A. editor. Parrot behavior. Ames (IA): Blackwell Publishing; 2006. p. 247–53.
7. Romagnano A. Reproduction and pediatrics. In: Harcourt-Brown N, Chitty J, editors. BSAVA manual of psittacine birds. 2nd edition. Cheltenham (UK): BSAVA; 2005. p. 222–33.
8. Romer L, editor. Cassowary husbandry manual, 1997. Currumbin Sanctuary. Available at: http://www.aszk.org.au/husbandry.bird.ews. Accessed February 15, 2012.
9. Romagnano A. Avian obstetrics. Semin Avian Exotic Pet Med 1996;5:180–8.
10. Romagnano A. Examination and preventive medicine protocols in psittacines. Vet Clin North Am 1999:22:333–55.
11. Rundel R. The Sonoma Bird Farm. Cassowary Husbandry Workshop. Available at: http://www.cassowary.com/workshop.html. Accessed February 15, 2012.

Nondomestic Avian Pediatric Pathology

Judy St. Leger, DVM, DACVP

KEYWORDS

- Avian • Pediatrics • Hand rearing • Neonatal • Nestling
- Chick • Pathology

INTRODUCTION

Chicks are not merely smaller versions of adult birds. Many diseases of avian neonates are unique to, or at least distinctive from the conditions of older birds. Because of small size, limited reserves, high requirements for growth, and developing immune status, diseases of chicks are more likely to result in death. Indeed, as babies age, the likelihood of any particular malady resulting in the death of the chick decreases. The improved survivability of older chicks and adults reflects both the success of medical intervention and the development of the immune system and general robustness of the chick. We will review the health concerns of non-domestic avian neonates with a goal of answering the question, "What is the lesion"? This will facilitate an overview of avian pediatric concerns and provide a road map of diagnosing those concerns.

INCUBATION

Even before chicks exit the egg, factors of incubation may contribute to health challenges. Incubation concerns can lead to failure to hatch, incomplete hatch, or hatching of weak and unthrifty chicks. A variety of issues related to breeder management and incubation can impact hatchability and chick survivability. Hatchability can be impacted by parental fitness as well as by such basic factors as formation of proper pairs. Nonbonded pairs can be as ineffective as same-sex pairs when it comes to producing fertile eggs. While these considerations do not impact chick health, they certainly are associated with reduced hatchability. A study by Cooper[1] reviews breeder vitamin and mineral imbalances and deficiencies that can reduce egg production and hatchability in ratites. Specific changes in the avian embryo associated with nutritional deficiencies in the parents include vitamin A deficiency associated with fetal malformations; vitamin D, niacin, and biotin deficiencies associated with fetal soft bones or bone and beak malformations; and

The author has nothing to disclose.
SeaWorld San Diego, 500 SeaWorld Drive, San Diego, CA 92109, USA
E-mail address: Judy.St.leger@seaworld.com

Vet Clin Exot Anim 15 (2012) 233–250
http://dx.doi.org/10.1016/j.cvex.2012.03.005
1094-9194/12/$ – see front matter © 2012 Published by Elsevier Inc.

parental iodine deficiency associated with incomplete abdominal closure. Many embryonic lesions are never tied to a specific etiology. But these examples suggest that full evaluation of breeder nutrition may identify the causes of many developmental concerns.

Embryonic mortality or cessation of development can result from improper incubation temperatures or humidity as well as excessive fluctuations in these parameters. Positional issues with hatching are addressed in this issue of the journal in an article by Rideout. High relative incubation humidity has been associated with embryonic anasarca and myopathy in hatchling ostrich chicks.[2] The myopathy reported specifically impacted hatchability due to damage to the muscles of the neck associated with pipping. Concerns of incubation impact can be evaluated by egg/embryo necropsy exams. These exams and the significance of various findings are presented in the associated article in this issue by Rideout.

Shell contamination with fecal material, dirt, and debris can allow entry of bacterial agents into the environment of the developing embryo. The developing avian embryo is separated from the general environment by a thin cuticle overlying the shell, a porous shell, and internal egg membranes. This cuticle can be compromised with abrasion or cleaning agents. The thousands of shell pores allow penetration of bacteria to the shell membranes. While shell pore densities vary, the bottom line is that the cuticle, egg shell, and internal membranes are good but not fool-proof protection for the embryo from infectious agents.[3] Rough egg handling during incubation can negatively impact the embryo. Excessive handling and jarring of eggs while turning, especially during the first week, may be harmful.

YOLK SAC ISSUES

During incubation, the yolk sac provides nutritional support for the developing avian embryo. Throughout most of avian embryonic development, the yolk is exterior to the body. From 2 to 4 days prior to hatch, the yolk sac is internalized and the abdominal wall of the chick closes to produce a small "umbilicus." The internalized yolk is absorbed slowly over the days following hatch and often can be seen in normal chicks as the outpocketing of the small intestine known as Merkel's diverticulum.[4]

Failure to internalize the yolk sac, often with a significant defect in the abdominal wall, is sometimes encountered in chicks. As with many developmental issues, this condition can be very mild with a small amount of the yolk sac remaining exterior to the body wall or severe with complete failure of internalization (**Fig. 1**). The condition can be corrected with surgical intervention if the problem is limited in scope and identified soon after hatching. Often, the condition is associated with a variety of concurrent developmental concerns and the death of the chick results. While published descriptions of this condition are limited,[5,6] many species demonstrate issues with internalization of yolk sac.

A retained yolk sac is a more frequent yolk sac abnormality than failure to internalize (**Fig. 2**). In this condition, the yolk sac is properly internalized but the yolk material is not absorbed over time. Altricial species use the yolk faster than do precocial birds. For example, starlings (*Sturnus vulgaris*) will absorb their yolk in 4 days, whereas the ostrich requires 8 or more days. Yolk sac absorption can be impacted by incubation temperature and humidity as well as chick feeding patterns; alterations in these factors may predispose birds to this condition. The presence of a yolk sac in any species beyond 13 days of age is sufficient criteria for the diagnosis of a retained yolk sac.[4]

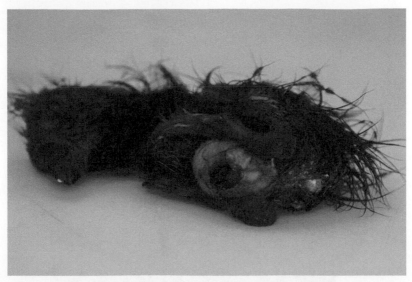

Fig. 1. Body as a whole, showing incomplete yolk internalization and closure of the umbilicus in a tufted puffin chick.

Affected chicks generally present anywhere from 5 to 15 days of age with a decreased appetite, lethargy, abdominal swelling, difficulty walking, dyspnea, and dehydration.[4] This is one of the major causes of mortality in ratite chicks less than 2 weeks of age.[7] A variety of waterfowl species and penguins also suffer significant neonatal mortalities from retained yolk sacs. Without surgical correction, the chicks often die. Gross findings include a large yolk sac present in a chick where involution should have reduced the structure to a vestigial body. The retained yolk content is typically watery. Culture of the yolk is indicated but the finding of sterile content within the yolk sac is not uncommon. Histology is unremarkable. Failure of yolk sac absorption can occur secondary to *Escherichia coli* septicemia (see **Fig. 2**). In these cases, *E coli* is commonly cultured from the yolk material. This condition is separate from primary omphalitis.[7]

Omphalitis is an infection of the yolk sac. This condition can easily extend to septicemia and the death of the chick. Yolk material is a rich medium for bacterial growth. Bacteria and parasites can gain access to the yolk itself via egg contamination, dirty incubation environments, or the umbilical wound (**Fig. 3**). *E coli, Proteus* sp, *Streptococcus faecalis,* and *Clostridium* sp were the agents most commonly isolated from yolk sac cultures performed in cases of yolk issues at the Denver Zoo.[4] In squab, infections of the yolk sac can occur from trichomoniasis. These chicks have very large retained and inflamed yolk sacs that compromise 20% to 40% of the chick's weight.[5]

Yolk sac infection is an important cause of death in juvenile bustards, being responsible for the deaths of 60% of houbara bustards, 25% of rufous-crested bustards, and 10% of kori bustards.[8] *Staphylococcus aureus* contamination of an incubator and high incubation humidity were responsible for the high incidence of yolk ac infection and septicemias in newly hatched houbara bustards in the 1994 breeding season.[8]

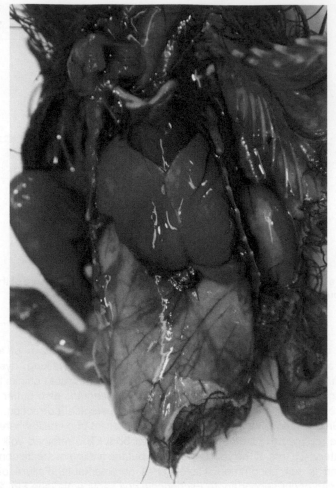

Fig. 2. Open coelom, showing retained yolk sac in a tufted puffin chick. Failure of umbilical closure promotes omphalitis and retained yolk sac.

CONGENITAL MALFORMATIONS/DEVELOPMENTAL ISSUES

Differentiation of congenital, developmental, genetic, and nutritional etiologies for deformities of avian neonates is very difficult. When studies in poultry or farmed nondomestic species have been performed, a few concrete causal relationships have been defined. This is not the case for most degenerative conditions of the avian neonate. Because of this, these conditions will be considered as a group. It is my desire that students looking to advance avian medicine consider evaluations that might improve our understanding of the cause-and-effect relationships of the etiologies for these conditions.

Congenital cardiac defects have been reported in an umbrella cockatoo (*Cacatua alba*) with a ventricular septal defect and persistent truncus arteriosus. A Mollucan cockatoo (*Cacatua moluccensis*) has been reported with a subvalvular septal defect and aortic hypoplasia.[9] A juvenile Houbara bastard (*Clamydotis undulate macqueenii*)

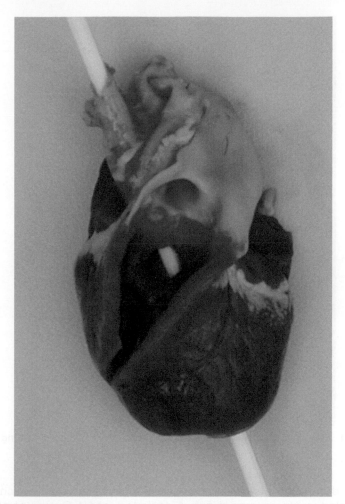

Fig. 3. Heart, showing congenital ventricular septal defect in a macaroni penguin. Death in this case was associated with marked pulmonary edema.

with sudden death demonstrated a ventricular septal defect at postmortem examination.[10] Ventricular septal defects have been seen in captive penguins with death from cardiac failure (see **Fig. 3**).

Developmental beak issues are common concerns in psittacine neonates. Scissor beak is a lateral deviation of the rhinotheca. It is a developmental abnormality that occurs most commonly in cockatoos and macaws. This is a problem usually limited to incubator-raised, hand-fed chicks. Because of this, proposed etiologies include improper temperature during incubation, genetics, nutrition, or incorrect feeding techniques. Mandibular prognathism occurs when the tip of the rhinotheca rests on or inside the gnatotheca. This developmental abnormality is most commonly seen in cockatoos (**Fig. 4**). The cause of this condition is unknown and may include genetics, improper incubation, and hand-feeding techniques. It is rarely seen in parent-raised birds. It is thought that when parent birds hook onto the chick's rhinotheca during feeding, they promote

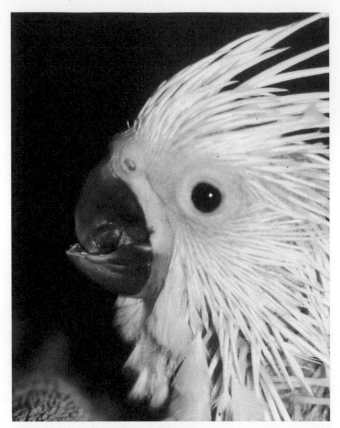

Fig. 4. Head, showing mandibular prognathism in an umbrella cockatoo nestling.

the normal development of the chick's beak. Congenital atresia of the choana has been reported in African gray chicks, 1 cockatoo, and 1 Quaker parakeet with unilateral choanal atresia.[11] The conditions were described with no concurrent craniofacial deformities.

Two cases of unilateral micromelia were described in wild juvenile little penguins (*Eudyptula minor*). In both cases, the left flipper was reduced in length and radiography demonstrated severe shortening and dysplasia of the humerus. One bird was underweight (0.55 kg) but otherwise in good condition. This bird also had shortening and fusion of the ulna, radius, metacarpals, and phalanges. The furcula was asymmetrical because the left clavicle was slightly thinner and more radiolucent than the right and was also slightly deviated to the right side.[12]

A variety of leg deformities or developmental issues are seen in avian neonates. Again, the etiologies are generally unknown but may reflect issues in nutrition, management, and genetics. Splay leg (spraddle leg) is a deformity in which one or both legs may deviate laterally, often from the stifle joint. A similar syndrome is seen in poultry and is called chondrodystrophy. Splay leg in psittacines is often attributed to substrate that does not provide good footing or trauma. Dietary imbalances such as metabolic bone disease have also been implicated. Stifle subluxation can occur due to disruption of the cruciate and/or collateral ligaments.

INFECTIOUS AND PARASITIC DISEASES

Infectious diseases are especially important in neonatal medicine and pathology because of the limited immune function of nestling birds. While all age classes are exposed to many of the same pathogens, it is often neonates that selectively demonstrate disease due to their lower resistance. The infective agent, as well as age at exposure, is important in determining disease manifestations. Often gross and histologic findings are nonspecific. In these cases, bacterial cultures and molecular investigations to confirm suspect viruses are critical to define the etiology.

The viruses of greatest concern due to associated death are the avian polyomavirus (APV), the circoviruses, and adenovirus. Avipox viruses impact many avian species and infections predominate in the immune-incompetent neonates. These infections are often more of a clinical nuisance than a fatal concern, but they certainly represent a condition of neonatal concern.

APV infections have been described for many years. These infections are generally classified as budgerigar fledgling disease and APV infection. The latter refers to infections of non-budgerigar psittacine species. Budgerigar death from APV is confined to nestlings between 10 and 25 days of age. Clinically, there is a sudden increase in the number of dead budgerigar nestlings in the nest boxes. At gross exam, birds are found to be stunted, often with abnormal feather development, skin discoloration, abdominal distension, ascites, hepatomegaly with parenchymal mottling, and occasional areas of hemorrhage. Microscopic examination reveals acute tissue necrosis and virus inclusions in the liver, spleen, kidney, feather follicles, skin, esophagus, brain, and heart. The virus can cause necrosis of neurons of the cerebellum; these birds show clinical head tremors. Chicks developing clinical signs after 15 days of often show bilaterally symmetrical dystrophic flight, tail, contour, and down feathering. This presentation is known as French molt; affected birds are called runners or creepers. This infection must be differentiated from psittacine beak and feather disease (PBFD).

Nonbudgerigar psittacines are also susceptible to APV infection. Disease in these birds occurs at different ages in different species. In conures, deaths typically occur in birds less than 6 weeks of age. Deaths in macaws and eclectus parrots occur in birds 14 weeks and younger. Infected nestlings appear healthy, show few premonitory signs, and then die acutely. Observant owners may notice delayed crop emptying, weakness, a generalized pallor, or bruising under the skin in the preceding hours before death. Necropsy findings commonly include generalized pallor with subcutaneous and subserosal hemorrhage, enlargement of the spleen and liver, and pericardial effusion and/or ascites (**Figs. 5** and **6**). Microscopic examination of the tissues reveals extensive areas of necrosis in the liver. Virus inclusion bodies are found in the spleen, mesangial cells of the kidney, and Kupffer cells of the liver. Necrosis of splenic cells is often massive. Less commonly, virus inclusions are found in other organ systems including the feather follicles. Occasionally, immune complexes are deposited within the glomerular tufts resulting in a membranous glomerulonephritis related to this infection (**Fig. 7**).

Avian circoviruses have been identified in an increasing array of species. While PBFD is the classic condition, closely related viral infections are seen in various species including pigeons and doves, canaries and finches, gulls, corvids, and ratites.[13–15] The characteristic lesions of PBFD have been well described and are similar to those seen in other species.[13,16] Feather changes associated with viral replication within feather follicles are easily identified, but it is the immunosuppressive actions of the virus that can kill. Feather lesions can occur without changes in

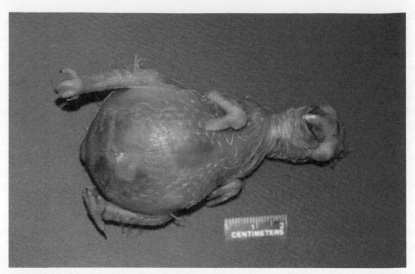

Fig. 5. Body as a whole, showing ascites in a young hand-fed macaw chick with APV.

lymphoid organs and vice versa. In many cases, feather lesions and lymphoid organ changes occur together.

The dermal form in fledgling birds is visible during feather formation after replacement of the neonatal down. Chicks as young as 2 months demonstrate feather necrosis, fracture and bending, hemorrhage, or premature shedding of developing feathers. The general appearance is of a bird with an extended pin feather phase, with patchy feather loss and deformed feathers (**Figs. 8** and **9**). Chicks that develop infection later in the feather formation cycle demonstrate a milder form of the disease. Characteristic botryoid deeply basophilic inclusions can be seen within the follicular epithelium often admixed with areas of necrosis and variable inflammatory infiltrates.

In lymphoid-focused cases in young birds, avian circoviruses present as depression, anorexia, crop stasis, and diarrhea followed by death in nestlings. This clinical presentation is particularly common in cases of PBFD in young cockatoos, African greys, and lovebirds. Gross lesions are nonspecific and often reflect secondary bacterial, viral, and fungal infections in addition to changes due to the virus. The major histologic changes of circoviral infection are commonly limited to the primary and secondary lymphoid tissues. These changes range from lymphofollicular hyperplasia to severe lymphoid necrosis and depletion. Lesions are common in the bursa of Fabricius and thymus and generally less severe in the spleen. As with the dermal form of the disease, characteristic intracytoplasmic inclusions are present within lymphocytes, macrophages, and epithelial cells.[13,16] Intracytoplasmic inclusions are more common in the spleen.

Circoviruses are not selective for feathers versus lymphoid organs. Indeed, a majority of infections likely involve both systems. An excellent example of avian circoviruses impacting both feathers and lymphoid organs has been reported in geese. A runting syndrome associated with a feathering disorder was reported in young geese from a commercial flock during a 9-week rearing period. Increased mortality was distributed evenly throughout the rearing period. Histology revealed lymphoid depletion and histiocytosis with basophilic inclusions within the bursa of Fabricius, spleen, and thymus.[13]

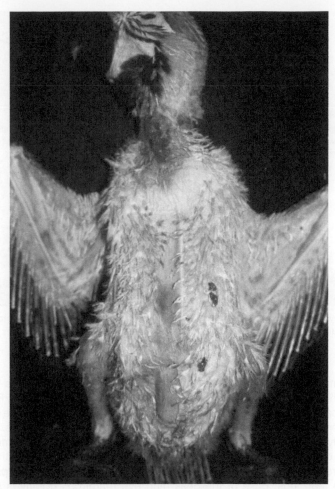

Fig. 6. Body as a whole, showing subcutaneous bruising in a blue and gold macaw due to APV.

A fatal adenoviral infection has impacted nestlings from several falcon species. Reports include neonatal Northern aplomado (*Falco femoralis septentrionalis*), peregrine (*Falco peregrinus anatum*), taita (*Falco fasciinucha*), and hybrid falcon nestlings. Nestlings generally showed lethargy and anorexia for 4 to 5 days prior to death. Gross examinations revealed congested lungs and mildly enlarged livers and spleens. Histologic review demonstrated acute necrotizing hepatitis and a nonsuppurative interstitial nephritis. Some birds demonstrate lymphoid depletion of the bursa of Fabricius. An acute necrotizing splenitis demonstrated intranuclear inclusion bodies within the splenic macrophages. Intranuclear inclusion bodies were also present in hepatocytes and in the renal tubular epithelial cells. Species differences are suggested for viral inclusion body locations.[17,18]

Avipox viral infections are a common concern in young birds. The conditions generally present with a benign cutaneous proliferation. These proliferations can impede feeding or become secondarily infected to promote death. In some cases, a

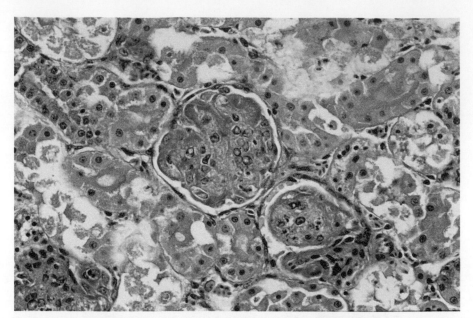

Fig. 7. Kidney photomicrograph (×10 magnification, PAS stain). Membranous glomerulonephritis in a sun conure associated with expansion of the glomerular tuft in cases of APV.

fatal systemic diphtheritic infection can occur. Approximately 60 free-living bird species representing about 20 families have been reported with avian pox. Psittacines are not typical hosts but Amazon parrots seem overrepresented with these infections. Many passerine species are regularly impacted by canary pox infections. Infections are generally thought to be transmitted by biting insects, specifically mosquitoes. Spread via contaminated surfaces such as perching material and bird feeders is reported. Gross lesions of the cutaneous presentation are focal, irregular proliferative changes on feet, legs, base of the beak, and eye margin. Histology is diagnostic demonstrating epithelial proliferation with abundant cytoplasmic eosinophilic inclusions along with variable dermal inflammation and areas of ulceration. The diphtheritic form appears as moist, fibrinonecrotic pseudomembrane of the mucus membranes of the mouth, respiratory, and upper digestive tracts. Histology again shows epithelial proliferation, but in these cases, significant necrosis and acute inflammation accompany the proliferations.[16]

Candida albicans is present in low levels in the normal avian oral mucosa. In situations of antibiotic administration, malnutrition, stress, or immunosuppression, *Candida* can proliferate and result in clinical disease. It is the most common fungal infection in the young bird and can result in thickening of the crop mucosa. This condition is often associated with delayed crop emptying or crop stasis. Associated with this condition, the crop contents often coagulate and present with a sour or fetid odor associated with overgrowth of yeast and bacteria.

Grossly, the crop wall is diffusely thickened by a white-tan pseudomembrane that follows the crop contours. In severe cases the crop mucosa takes on a "Turkish towel appearance" (**Fig. 10**). This proliferation gives the crop a doughy and distended feel on palpation. Histologically, there is a fibrinous pseudomembrane with abundant budding yeast and pseudohyphae extending through the mucosa. Inflammation is

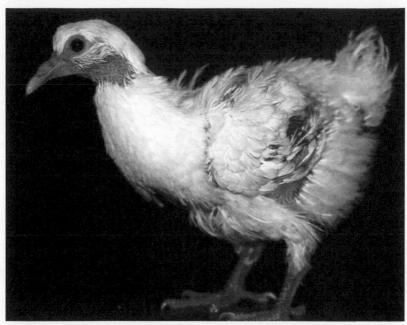

Fig. 8. Body as a whole, showing wing, tail, and scattered body feather dystrophy and loss in a squab due to columbiforme circovirus infection. These birds died from the associated lymphoid necrosis and secondary bacterial and fungal infections.

variable, but a mild to moderate heterophilic infiltrate in the crop mucosa and submucosa is not uncommon.

Aspergillosis is a condition of concern for all avian patients. It is of particular significance to sea birds and to neonates. The infections typically involve the respiratory tract and vary from focal tracheitis to more diffuse airsacculitis to fulminant pneumonia, often with associated changes in the other components of the respiratory tract. Gross examination can reveal focal tracheal plugs, multifocal tan nodules within the lungs or air sacs, and thick, firm sheets or distinct luminal masses composed of inflammatory debris and fungal hyphae (**Fig. 11**). Histologically, inflammation has a granulomatous character often with giant cells. Fungal hyphae tend to be in areas with better aeration. Vasoinvasion is common.

A recent study by Olias and colleagues[19] demonstrates fungal pneumonia as a major cause of mortality in white stork (*Ciconia ciconia*) chicks. The percentage of affected lung tissue varied from 10% to approximately 80% of the lung parenchyma. In this investigation, they identified invasive fungal pneumonia in the lungs of 45 (44.6%) from 101 examined white stork nestlings as a major infectious cause in mortality prior to fledging. Overall, *A fumigatus* was detected in 57.9% of the positive cases and was involved in 71.4% cases of severe fungal pneumonia.

Bacterial sepsis is a major concern in baby birds. The incompletely developed immune system and immunosuppressive viruses make bacterial infections a more serious concern in neonates compared to adults. Common portals of entry include the umbilicus and yolk sac (omphalitis), as well as the gastrointestinal and respiratory tracts. The agents of greatest concern are similar to those in adult birds. They include *E coli*, *Klebsiella*, *Salmonella* sp, *Pseudomonas* sp, and *Chlamydophilia* sp. The

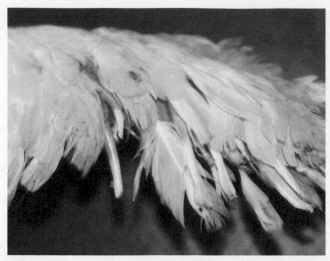

Fig. 9. Skin, wing, showing close-up view of feather dystrophy demonstrating clubbed, fractured, and misshapen feathers from columbiforme circoviral infection.

conditions present exactly as with older birds. However, incompletely developed immune function makes these a common cause of avian neonatal mortality.

"Lockjaw syndrome" is a specific clinical entity in neonatal cockatiels. The condition is generally associated with infection by *Bordetella avium,* but a variety of bacterial agents have been isolated from cases. Some reported cases have had *Chlamydophilia psittaci* as a coinfection associated with *B avium.* The condition is characterized by inability to articulate the temporomandibular joint and open the beak. Patients are typically presented between 2 to 4 weeks of age. Grossly, chicks have a mild nasal discharge and a mildly swollen head. The jaw is fused shut and cannot be opened with moderate pressure.[20] Histologically, there is a necrotizing rhinitis and sinusitis, as well as myositis, perineuritis, and osteomyelitis affecting the jaw muscles and cranial bones. The myositis is extensive and often associated with marked fibrosis. This change, along with a fibrosing temperomandibulitis, is responsible for the jaw immobility.[21] Inoculation studies suggest that birds exposed after 30 days of age developed either mild or no clinical disease.[20]

Ornithobacterium rhinotracheale has been associated with respiratory infections and mortality in nestling falcons from a large falcon breeding farm. In a group of 40 nestlings, 10 birds demonstrated respiratory distress and 3 died from infection. Postmortem examination demonstrated a severe serofibrinous exudate in the air sacs. Histopathologic review revealed a severe acute fibrinous airsacculitis, visceral pleuritis, and focal necrosis in the spleen with lymphocytic depletion. No older nestlings or adult birds demonstrated illness during this event. The source of the infection is presumed to be infected poultry provided as food items in combination with inclement weather resulting in nestling chilling.[22]

MANAGEMENT CONCERNS

Chilling is a common concern in commercial poultry but is underrespected when it comes to nondomestic species. While not a disease in itself, chilling such as is seen during periods of rainy, wet weather for birds reared in the nest can add stress and

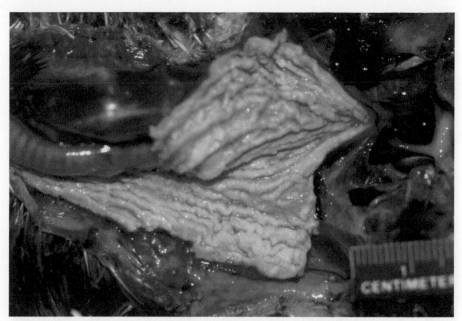

Fig. 10. Crop mucosa, showing diffuse thickening of the crop mucosa in an Amazon parrot with ingluvitis from a *Candida* sp infection.

promote disease development. There are no specific associated gross or histologic findings with this condition. However, when instances of disease seem to impact a greater number of chicks than expected, a review of environmental conditions may suggest chilling as a factor. Most hand-reared birds are maintained in temperature-controlled environments to minimize the possibilities of this stressor.

Damage to the crop is a common issue, especially in hand-fed babies. Uneven heating of formula with the formation of "hot spots" can result in mucosal burns and subsequent necrosis. These injuries can lead to localized cellulitis and subsequent sepsis or trauma can extend through the underlying skin to result in a fistula with local infection.[23]

Aspiration pneumonia is a common concern in both hand-fed and parent-reared chicks (**Fig. 12**). The condition can be associated with overfilling of the crop but is also seen with weak birds that regurgitate and subsequently aspirate. Deaths can occur from asphyxiation due to physical obstruction of the airway or via airsacculitis and pneumonia from secondary infections. The subacute condition typically results in a mixed bacterial infection and can lead to sepsis. Gross exam may demonstrate formula within air sacs and the major airways or an airsacculitis and multifocal pneumonia. Caution should be taken when evaluating tracheal formula to ensure that aspiration occurred antemortem and is not due to relaxation of the larynx after death.

Ingestion of foreign bodies is not uncommon as a gastrointestinal concern of young birds. In some cases, the chicks enthusiastically consume inappropriate materials such as bedding from their environment. In other cases, overanxious parents may actually provide nondigestible materials to chicks. I have experienced this in a number of toucan chick mortalities associated with parents feeding the chicks small sticks (**Fig. 13**). Foreign material can cause blockage, irritation, or perforation of the GI tract.

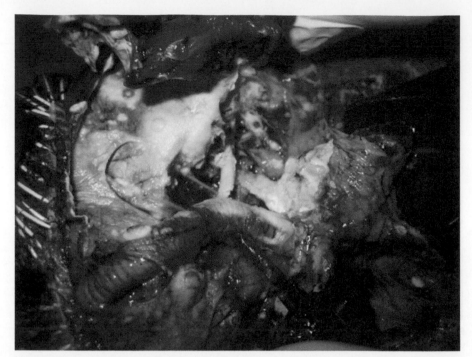

Fig. 11. Clavicular air sac at cardiac base, showing multifocal granulomas and fibrinous airsacculitis from aspergillosis in a young tufted puffin chick.

Constricted toe syndrome is a common nestling condition seen in macaws, African grey parrots, eclectus parrots, and cockatoos. Grossly, there is circumferential constriction of a digit with swelling of the distal portion of 1 or more toes. If left untreated, the condition results in avascular necrosis of the digit tips due to the constriction.[24]

NUTRITIONAL ISSUES

Hepatic lipidosis is a specific disease of concern in hand-fed cockatoos and, rarely, macaws. Moluccan and umbrella cockatoos are overrepresented in these cases. The birds present between 3 and 10 weeks of age with distention of the abdominal wall to accommodate the enlarged liver. On direct exam, the liver is enlarged, friable, and pale with rounded edges and often with associated hemorrhage. Histologically, there is diffuse hepatocellular lipidosis and some degree of disorganization of the liver architecture. These cases typically have a history of feeding cockatoo babies a hand-feeding formula that is higher in fat than recommended. This alteration can be achieved either by adding fat such as peanut butter or oils to prepared diets or feeding handfeeding formula designed for macaws. This formulation has higher lipid content than standard formulations. When fed to cockatoo babies, these high-fat diets produce hepatic lipidosis that can progress to death.[5]

Stunting is a pathologic concern that typically occurs within the first month of life for psittacines. The condition is a nonspecific reflection of poor growth rate. The underlying condition is poor growth due to husbandry, malnutrition, inadequate feeding (volume, frequency, or nutritional density of food), or illness. Stunting can

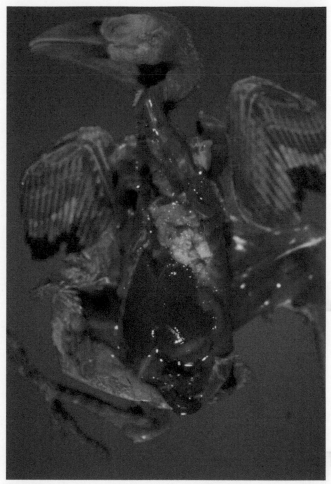

Fig. 12. Lung, showing aspiration pneumonia in a 25-day tocanet. This is a case of extensive bacterial pneumonia. Death from this condition can result from asphyxiation or secondary airsacculitis and pneumonia.

be associated with inexperienced hand-feeders.[5] Stunted birds are thin and often dehydrated. The head is disproportionately large as compared with the body. Eye and ear opening may be delayed. The delayed ear opening is sometimes associated with development of otitis externa. Swirling abnormal feathering patterns may develop on the head of a stunted chick.

PARASITIC CONDITIONS

Red mites (*Dermanyus gallinae*) and northern fowl mites (*Ornytisluss sylvarium*) can infest nest boxes and parasitize chicks. Chicks are often quiet and fluffed. They may die in the nest with no specific gross lesions.[6] On internal examination, organs may appear generally pale due to blood loss. Commonly, there are no significant histologic changes associated with these concerns. The diagnosis is best made by direct examination of the nest box. In areas where fire ants are present, these insects

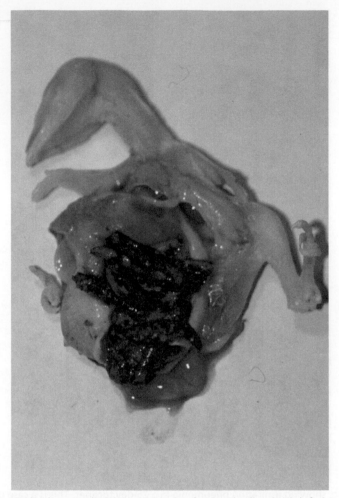

Fig. 13. Ventricular lumen, showing ventricular foreign bodies (sticks) fed to a nestling collared aracari by parents. Young birds can obtain GI foreign bodies by parental feeding and indiscriminant ingestion of environmental materials.

present another potential cause of chick mortality with no significant gross or histologic changes. Infestation of the nest box or nest log with fire ants can cause direct damage to the chicks by the effects of stings as well as deterring parents from rearing responsibilities. Unlike with mites, it is much more likely that fire ants will remain on the dead chick for identification. Because of this, do not discount ant invasion of chicks as a benign postmortem event. Identification of the invading ant species is may suggest a diagnosis.

Coccidiosis is generally considered a condition of the gastrointestinal tract in adult birds. Infections are acquired by exposure to contaminated environments. However, in both free ranging and captive crane species, *Eimeria* spp infections in chicks can become widely disseminated.[6] These infections result in the death of gruiforme chicks. Infection is similar to the adult route of environmental exposure. However, overwhelming exposure produces extensive disseminated disease. Clinical presentations can vary from progressive weakness, emaciation, greenish diarrhea, dyspnea, and recumbency to sudden death. Gross examination reveals nodules within trachea, lungs, air sacs, heart, liver, spleen, and intestines. Areas of acute congestion and hemorrhage are evident in the lungs and liver. Histologically, the nodules are granulomatous inflammation with merozoites contained within macrophages. There is a moderate concurrent nonsuppurative vasculitis throughout the body.[25]

SUMMARY

This is a snapshot of avian neonatal pathology—not an exhaustive review. Through knowledge and recognition of the significant pathogenic challenges of avian neonates and the associated lesions, avian practitioners can improve their diagnostic and therapeutic success. An area of need for avian research is determining the specific pathogenesis of many conditions affecting avian neonates. By narrowing the specific etiologies, we can improve management and reduce neonatal concerns.

REFERENCES

1. Cooper RG. Handling, incubation, and hatchability of ostrich (Struthio camelus var. domesticus) eggs: a review. J Appl Poult Res 2001;10:262–73.
2. Philbey AW, Button C, Geister AW, et al. Anasarca and myopathy in ostrich chicks. Aust Vet J 1991;68:237–40.
3. Tung MA, Garland ME, Gill PK. A scanning election microscope study of bacterial invasion in the hen's egg shell. J Inst Can Sci Techol Aliment 1991;12:16–22.
4. Kenny D, Cambre RC. Indications and technique for the surgical removal of the avian yolk sac. J Zoo Wildl Med 1992;23(1):55–61.
5. Flammer K, Clubb SL. Neonatology. In: Ritchie BW, Harrison GI, Harrison LR, editors. Avian medicine: principles and application. Lake Worth (FL): Wingers Publishing; 1994. p. 805–40.
6. Carpenter JW. Gruiformes (cranes, limpkins, rails, gallinules, coots, bustards). In: Fowler ME, editor. Zoo and wildlife medicine. 5th edition. Philadelphia: WB Saunders; 2003. p. 171–9.
7. Dzoma B, Dorrestein G. Yolk sac retention in the Ostrich (Struthio camelus): Histopathologic, anatomic, and physiologic considerations. J Avian Med Surg 2001;15: 81–9.
8. Bailey TA, Nicholls PK, Samour JH, et al. Postmortem findings in bustards in the United Arab Emirates. Avian Dis 1996;40(2):296–305.
9. Evans DE, Tully TN Jr, Strickland KN, et al. Congenital cardiovascular anomalies, including ventricular septal defects, in 2 cockatoos. J Avian Med Surg 2001;15(2): 101–6.
10. Bailey TA, Kinne J. Ventricular septal defect in Houbara bustard (Clamydotis undulate macqueenii). Avian Dis 2001;45:229–33.
11. Greenacre CB, Watson E, Ritchie BW. Choanal atresia in an Africa grey parrot and an umbrella cockatoo. J Assoc Avian Vets 1993;7(1):19–22.
12. Raidal SR, Shearer PL, Cannell BL, et al. Micromelia in little penguins (Eudyptula minor). J Avian Med Surg 2006;20(4):258–62.
13. Woods LW, Lattimer KS. Circovirus infection of nonpsittacine birds. J Avian Med Surg 2000;14:154–63.
14. Twentyman CM, Alley MR, Meers J, et al. Circovirus-like infection in a southern black-backed gull (Larus dominicanus). Avian Pathol 1999;28:513–6.
15. Stewart ME, Perry R, Raidal SR. Identification of a novel circovirus in Australian ravens (Corvus coronoides) with feather disease. Avian Pathol 2006;35:86–92.

16. Ritchie BW. Viruses. In: Ritchie BW Harrison GJ, Harrison LR, editors. Avian medicine: principles and application. Lake Worth (FL): Wingers Publishing; 1994. p. 888–94.

17. Van Wettere AJ, Wunschmann A, Latimer KS, et al. Adenovirus infection in Taita falcons (Falco fasciinucha) and hybrid falcons (Falco rusticolus x Falco peregrinus). J Avian Med Surg 2005;19(4):280–5.

18. Oaks JL, Schrenzel M, Rideout B, et al. Isolation and epidemiology of falcon adenovirus. J Clin Microbiol 2005;43(7):3414–20.

19. Olias P, Gruber A, Winfried B, et al. Fungal pneumonia as a major cause of mortality in white stork (Ciconia ciconia) chicks. Avian Dis 2010;54:94–8.

20. Clubb SL, Homer BL, Pisani J, et al. Outbreaks of bordetellosis in psittacines and ostriches. In: Proceedings of the Association of Avian Veterinarians. Reno (NV), September 28–30, 1994. Madison (WI): Omnipress; 1994. p. 63–8.

21. Fitzgerald SD, Hanika C, Reed WM. Lockjaw syndrome in cockatiels associated with sinusitis. Avian Pathol 2001;30(1):49–53.

22. Hafez H, Lierz M. Ornithobacterium rhinotracheale in nestling falcons. Avian Dis 2010;54:161–3.

23. Clubb SL, Wolf S, Phillips A. Psittacine pediatric medicine. In: Schubot RM, Clubb KJ, Clubb SL, editors. Psittacine aviculture: perspectives, techniques and research. Loxahatchee (FL): Avicultural Breeding and Research Center; 1992.

24. Clipsham R, Noninfectious diseases of pediatric psittacines. Semin Avian Exotic Pet Med 1992:1:22–33.

25. Novilla MN, Carpenter JW. Pathology and pathogenesis of disseminated visceral coccidiosis in cranes. Avian Pathol 2010;33(3):275–80.

Reptilian and Amphibian Pediatric Medicine and Surgery

Jay D. Johnson, DVM

KEYWORDS

- Reptile • Amphibian • Pediatric • Juvenile • Medicine
- Surgery

Pediatrics medicine and surgery, as a discipline of human medicine, encompasses care of infants, children, and adolescents. In the field of herpetological medicine and surgery, it covers the neonates, juveniles, and subadults. For reptiles and amphibians, this period has a variability of as little as a few months to 20 years or more depending on the species. Several different types of parental care and behavior have been observed in a wide variety of reptiles and amphibians, including crocodilians, some skinks, some monitors, salamanders, some frogs, and a few other species. However, the offspring of most reptilian and amphibian species are on their own for survival from the time of birth or hatching.

Reptilian and amphibian pediatric medicine and surgery can be challenging. In addition to knowing the principles of herpetological medicine and surgery, veterinarians must know the individual species' diet and husbandry requirements and further understand differences between neonates, juveniles, and adults. There are often differences in husbandry and dietary requirements between juveniles and adults of the same species. Some of these differences are general across broad species groups, while others may be specific to an individual species. Understanding these differences is important for assessing history, identifying problems originating from improper husbandry, identifying medical problems, and implementing proper treatment and care. Reptilian and amphibian pediatric patients can be very small, and the ability to perform complete diagnostic workups at the same level as for other larger vertebrates is challenging. Many diagnostic procedures can be performed with small sample sizes and the practitioner must be able to prioritize testing for each individual situation.

PEDIATRIC MEDICINE AND SURGERY

Understanding the individual species' biological ecology is important for providing proper care and assessment of problems. It is nearly impossible for a veterinarian to know all of this information. Often one must generalize across similar species or

The author has nothing to disclose.
Arizona Exotic Animal Hospital, 744 North Center Street, Mesa, AZ 85201, USA
E-mail address: jjohnson@azeah.com

Vet Clin Exot Anim 15 (2012) 251–264
doi:10.1016/j.cvex.2012.02.001
vetexotic.theclinics.com

similar groups and try to identify smaller individual differences. There are some general concepts that are useful to understand when assessing the history and care of reptiles.

Reptiles can be either viviparous (live birth) or oviparous (produce eggs). Most reptiles and amphibians are oviparous. Knowing the reproductive biology of the species you are working with is beneficial in assessing the history of a patient or case. Health problems and nutritional status of the mother can have significant effects on her offspring. Also, improper temperature or humidity conditions during egg incubation can lead to health problems for the offspring. Offspring can be immunocompromised and have increased risk for infection, have metabolic abnormalities, or have anatomical defects secondary to improper gestation. Many juveniles are exposed to pathogens and parasites of the adult (either directly or indirectly) that may or may not create illness depending on the health of the offspring. External anatomical defects are often visible to the practitioner but represent only a small portion of what can go wrong. Many problems associated with internal fetal development may not become apparent for weeks and even months after birth or hatching.

Examination

A thorough history needs to be obtained along with the physical examination. History items of importance for pediatrics include: What is the history of the parents (if known)? Where and when was the pet obtained? Is it housed alone, or are there others in the cage with it? Are there other reptiles at home? Are other reptiles at home ill? What cleaning and disinfection techniques are used (including products)? Is there any previous medical history? What is the caging/enclosure setup (be sure to include size, substrate, hiding options, high and low temperatures, humidity, lighting, ultraviolet [UV] access)? If a species that requires UV light, what type of bulb is used? How close is the bulb to the animal and when was the bulb last changed? What husbandry is performed? What is the diet (not only what is offered, but what does the animal actually eat)?

Initial visual examination should be performed to assess overall body condition, dermal coloration and condition, hydration, obvious lesions, and gross deformities. Gently hold and restrain the entire body when possible. Care must be used to prevent injury when handling juvenile reptiles. Tail sloughing and limb fractures can occur. Handle patients close to a table surface to prevent injury if they jump or fall. Perform the physical exam over a surface that will not absorb important diagnostic samples if the patient urinates or defecates during the physical exam. Use wet nonpowdered latex gloves when handling amphibians to prevent skin damage. Magnification devices can sometimes aid in visualization of abnormalities. The use of an otoscope magnification lens and lighting without a cone attached often aids in visual examination. Transillumination of some small reptiles and amphibians can be performed to identify gross internal problems.

Sex Determination

Although sex of a juvenile often does not have an impact on its health, many clients want to know the sex of their pet. This may be due to curiosity, a desire to not have to invest the time and money into a pet they may not want or be able to keep, or developing an emotional bond to pets they may not be able to maintain together and keep long term. Some clients want to know if they have a male and a female with future plans of breeding them. For some species, it can be difficult to maintain multiple males together. Some clients do not want to deal with reproduction and want to identify that they have juveniles that are the same sex before spending time and money on raising them up to adults. Most reptiles are not sexually dimorphic until puberty occurs. In the wild, puberty may occur in as little as a few months or as late as 15 to 20 years depending on the species. Puberty does not always coincide with the species reaching subadult to adult sizes. In captivity, many reptiles can grow in size at rates far faster than they achieve in the wild; in captivity, often puberty is achieved earlier than it would have occurred in the wild. There may be a period where captive "big babies," prepubescent adult-sized individuals without normal sexually dimorphic traits, are challenging to determine sex.

Most reptiles, other than snakes and viviparous lizards, have temperature-dependent sex determination during incubation. The species, temperatures, and times of effects are beyond the scope of this article, and often the information is unknown for most purchased as pets. However, several methods can be used to help assist in determination of sex.

In turtles and tortoises (Chelonia), differences in tail length, location of vent in relation to caudal aspect of the anal scutes, anal and gular scute conformation, and plastron conformation can become apparent between male and females as sexual dimorphism occurs. In box turtles, males often have red irises, while females often have brown, orange, or greenish irises. Endoscopic identification of gonad type is one of the most commonly used ways of confirm sex of juvenile chelonia when necessary. This requires the practitioner to have the appropriate equipment and knowledge of the procedure.[1,2]

For snakes, tail length and conformation can sometimes allow for a subjective determination of sex. Males often have thicker and longer tails than females. Lubricated snake sexing probes can be inserted into the vent, then passed caudally under the skin along the ventral tail. In females, probes should reach a depth of only 4 or 5 subcaudal scales, or less. In males, probes often exceed a depth of 6 subcaudal scales as they pass down one of the inverted hemipenes. Care should be taken not to injure the hemipenis while probing. With experience, digital manipulation of the base of the juvenile hemipenis can cause it to evert out through the vent. In some species of boas and pythons, there are "spurs" on either side of the vent. These spurs often grow larger in males than in females.

Early sex determination of lizards is very challenging. Many species have secretory glands along their ventral hind legs called femoral pores. These often grow larger in males as they approach puberty. In some species such as green iguanas and bearded dragons, paired hemipenis bulges can be seen on the ventral tail base caudal to the vent. Probing is often inaccurate and can result in hemipenis damage. Endoscopic identification of gonads can be performed. Often one must wait for color and/or anatomical changes associated with sexual dimorphism to occur to be able to determine the sex of most lizards.

Sex determination of amphibians is highly variable depending on the species. Some have only seasonal sexual dimorphism. Nuptial pads in a variety of locations on the body, enlarged toe pads, cloacal glands, color, size, and morphology may all aid in identification of sex depending on the species.

HUSBANDRY

Husbandry of juvenile reptiles and amphibians is often slightly different than adults of the same species. Juveniles of many species often live in different or smaller areas of their environments than adults to avoid predation, prevent dehydration, and find appropriate food. Environmental enrichment is important for proper development of normal behaviors. Stress and reluctance to move about the cage will impair proper thermoregulation, increase risk of disease, decrease foraging, and prevent proper growth.

Caging/Enclosures

Captive juvenile reptiles should be provided an environment mimicking their natural environment to minimize stress. Ground-dwelling reptiles should be provided one or more shelter/burrow/hiding areas. There should be plenty of items such as branches, rocks, and plants at ground level. Arboreal reptiles should be provided with several branch areas allowing basking and cooling. There should be leaves or other materials present to allow concealment. If live plants are used, make sure they are nontoxic for herbivorous reptiles. Artificial plants are not recommended for omnivorous and herbivorous reptiles as they may ingest them. Rocks and other heavy items should be placed directly on the floor of the enclosure to prevent burrowing reptiles from digging under them and becoming crushed. Juvenile amphibians need to have plenty of hiding areas in and out of the water depending on species and stage of development.

Many different types of substrates can be used, and the appropriateness of each varies depending on the species being housed. Substrates most resembling native environments are best. Substrates retaining moisture should be used for species that need it. Ingestion of and subsequent intestinal impaction from the substrate have been reported for most substrates. In my experience, it is not so much the substrate that is the problem as it is the way food is presented. Moist greens or vegetable items, small mice, and small insects should not be placed directly on the substrate. The substrate will often adhere to them and become ingested. Food items can be placed on plates or flat rocks or in bowls.

Humidity in many homes is very low due to air conditioning and heating. Additional heating of cages further decreases humidity within many cages. There is a significant difference in ground-level humidity and underground humidity, such as in burrows. Chronic low cage humidity often leads to some level of dehydration, even in desert species. Proper humidity should be maintained in the air for arboreal reptiles and amphibians and in the burrow/shelter areas of ground-dwelling reptiles and amphibians. To maintain proper air humidity, owners can use a spray bottle to mist the cage as needed or use commercially available misting or fogging systems. To maintain proper burrow/shelter humidity, moistened substrates such as peat or sphagnum moss can be placed in burrow/shelter areas and remoistened as needed to maintain necessary increased humidity in these areas. Inadequate humidity can lead to dehydration and improper development for some species. Excessive moisture can predispose some species to diseases of the integument and respiratory tract. A hygrometer should be used to monitor humidity levels in the cage.

Proper water quality, temperature, and pH are important for aquatic species. Simple test strips and kits made for testing fish tanks are available at most pet stores. Water quality should be checked routinely to identify water problems prior to subsequent secondary health issues occurring.

Diet

Many juveniles have increased protein and other nutritional requirements in comparison to adults of the same species. However, in the wild they still have to work for their food and food is not always available in the wild. In captive situations where food is readily available and provided frequently, overfeeding often occurs. Overfeeding can lead to obesity and improper development. Rapid growth may not be synonymous with good health.

Captive diets should be as close as possible to natural diets. Quick Internet searches or species reference books often can provide this information. Captive raised insects, produce from stores, and commercial diets often do not provide complete nutrition. Holding insects purchased and feeding them nutritious diets (gut loading) for a period of times, dusting food items with calcium, and dusting food items with other vitamin and mineral supplements may also be needed. For active insects such as crickets, gut loading is preferred because powders that are dusted on will quickly be removed as the insects groom. Only enough insects that can be consumed within a few hours should be placed in the cage. Some types of insects, if not eaten, may attack and feed on small or debilitated reptiles. Some herbivorous reptiles need bulk coarse fiber in their diets (grass, grass hay, and plant and tree leaves). Some omnivorous species eat higher proportions of animal or insect items as juveniles.

Nutritional analysis of items fed should also be considered. Desert reptile species that lack salt excretion glands manage potassium by precipitating it with urates. If systemic potassium levels are too high, it will cause the body to make and excrete more urates, creating a negative nitrogen balance and thus impairing growth and development. High-potassium diets can impair growth of some species. Some species have been shown to preferentially avoid diets high in potassium regardless of the protein content.[3]

Care must be taken when supplements are used. Excessive calcium is likely to not be absorbed and passed through the digestive tract. Oversupplementation with calcium and vitamin D_3 can lead to tissue mineralization and health problems later in life. Beta-carotenes are often used in supplements as a vitamin A precursor. Some species, such as leopard geckos, seem to not process beta-carotenes well and do better with supplements with vitamin A in them. Some species, such as chameleons, have a much higher requirement for vitamin A and need supplementation more frequently than other reptiles.

Some reptiles obtain the microorganisms required for proper digestion by eating dirt or copraphagy of adult feces. These reptile species often grow better and faster when this occurs. For many herbivorous reptiles, some dirt or feces from the parent or a healthy adult should be provided in the cage. Physical exams and fecal evaluations of adults should be performed before offering their feces or feces-contaminated soil to juveniles.

Thermoregulation

Many physiologic processes of reptiles are temperature dependent. Reptiles often require a range of temperatures to accomplish all of their necessary physiologic processes. It is important to provide the appropriate range of temperatures within caging/enclosures that will allow thermoregulation and completion of physiological processes necessary for growth and development. The Internet and many species-specific books can be good sources for finding proper temperature ranges. When this is not available, then one should consider the climate of the part of the world where the species naturally exists. One must also consider the specific part of its natural environment and associated microclimate it lives in. Enclosures should be constructed in ways that allow the reptile or amphibian to be comfortable moving though its captive environment to different temperature zones.

UV Lighting

Skin exposure to UVB lighting is required for proper photobiosynthesis of vitamin D_3 in many reptiles. Exposure to UVA lighting is necessary for many normal behaviors. Veterinarians should know the individual requirements for the species in question. In general, most chelonians and lizards require some exposure to UVB light. For species requiring it, a review of proper UVB light exposure should be carefully assessed with the owner. There is no regulation on efficacy of UVB lighting commercially produced for reptiles and there are significant differences between types and quality of bulbs available from different manufacturers. Visible light produced does not ensure UV light output. UV output from bulbs decreases with time. Due to the gradual decline in UV output from bulbs over time, growing reptiles and amphibians should have fluorescent UV lighting replaced with new bulbs every 6 months or if bulb failure is suspected. In most cases ground surface or basking areas should be within 18 inches of fluorescent bulb. Plastic or glass surfaces, unless UV transmissible, will block the beneficial UVB lighting from reaching the skin. Screen cage tops and sides of enclosures also block some UV light from reaching the patient. Always review cage setup and location of the UV lighting.

Mercury vapor and metal halide lamps produce the highest UV output and heat. This combination is advantageous for desert species that require more heat and spend more time basking naturally in the sun. They can create problems for small enclosures. Dermal burns can occur from over exposure to UV lighting, and cage overheating can occur. Skin neoplasia may also be associated with over exposure to UV light. It is important to match the type of bulb to the patient and the cage. Lower-intensity fluorescent bulbs are more appropriate for small cages and species that do not need a lot of basking time. Higher-intensity mercury vapor lamps should be used in larger cages or enclosures and for species that spend more time basking in hot environments.

If multiple juveniles are kept in the same cage, competition for basking areas can occur if multiple sites are not present. This can lead to UVB deficiency in the weaker or less dominant juveniles in the cage even when UV lighting is present.

When and where possible, exposure to natural sunlight is often very beneficial as it provides the optimum UV spectrum. One must consider the appropriateness of the local outdoor climate when deciding if it is appropriate to have pet reptiles outside. Outdoor enclosures need to allow the ability of the reptile or amphibian to move in and out of the sun as necessary depending on body temperatures attained. Sufficient ventilation and shade must be present to prevent overheating. Depending on the outdoor climate, enclosures may need to either insulate from cold weather or have a heat source depending on the species and time of year. Enclosures should also be constructed in ways that prevent escape and prevent harm from predation.

DIAGNOSTIC TESTING

Patient size and sample size can limit some diagnostic abilities. However, many diagnostic procedures can be performed successfully if care is taken to collect and preserve samples and then interpret them accurately.

Direct fecal evaluations can be performed on 0.01 mL of feces to diagnose intestinal parasites. Small numbers of intestinal parasites seen on direct microscopic examination of a drop of urine can indicate higher numbers present in feces. Fecal flotation can be performed when sample size permits. Impression and aspirate cytology can often aid in diagnostic workup. Volumes of 0.01 mL of blood can be used to make a blood smear to identify toxic changes in white blood cells and identify some blood parasites. Venipuncture sites are often the same locations used in adults, however needle sizes of 25 gauge or less are often necessary for use. Abaxis blood chemistry analyzers (Abaxis, Union City, CA, USA) can perform a reptilian plasma chemistry panel using small (100–120 μL) samples of whole blood or plasma. Microhematocrit tubes can be used to obtain hematocrits of small amounts of blood.

Some polymerase chain reaction (PCR) tests are available for reptilian pathogens. These tests can be performed on small sample sizes collected onto a cotton swab. Often PCR tests can be run using the same samples used for fecal testing and cytologies. Refer to individual labs' requirements for sample amount needed and proper processing. Dental radiograph machines can be very effective for images of small patients.

For identification of problems within a group in which in-hospital samples tested are not diagnostic, necropsy and histopathology can be very useful. Tissues, or often the whole body opened and preserved in formalin, should be sent to a laboratory with a pathologist familiar with reptiles and amphibians for best results. Some veterinary colleges will accept live animals mailed to them for initial exam, euthanasia, and necropsy.

MEDICAL PROBLEMS
Congenital Defects

Congenital defects can and do occur. Defects causing gross anatomical changes are easy to diagnose. Animals with some anatomical defects such as missing an eye, limb, or digit; abnormal scute patterns on the shell; and even 2 heads are sometimes able to survive. Segmental aplasia of the gastrointestinal (GI) tract, cardiovascular defects, and other visceral malformations and physiologic impairments may not be visible on exam. These individuals are often "poor doers" that do not feed or grow normally despite proper care and eventually die.

Developmental defects can and do occur. Some of these are related to nutrition and environmental factors and others may be associated with genetic abnormalities. Thorough evaluation of history and care needs to be assessed along with appropriate diagnostic workups before defaulting to an exclusional diagnosis of genetic disorder.

Yolk Sac Diseases

Yolk sacs are normally internalized into the body prior to hatching, then fully absorbed over a period of weeks to months after hatching. This gives many neonatal reptiles a nutrition source for a short period until they emerge from the ground and are foraging and feeding. Problems can occur where reptiles hatch or are born prior to yolk sac internalization. Without immediate correction, these exposed yolk sacs often rupture from trauma; infection ensues, followed by death. Internalized yolk sacs sometimes are not fully absorbed and end up serving as sequestrum of media for bacterial growth and infection.

Depending on the size of the opening into the coelomic cavity around the yolk sac, several treatment options can be used to correct nonresorbed yolk sacs. Patients with small exteriorized yolk sacs can be kept on soft moist substrate and monitored closely for trauma or signs of infection until the sac has resorbed naturally. Yolk sacs can also be surgically removed. The base of the sac should be cleaned with dilute povidine-iodine and a ligature placed at the base as close to its intestinal junction as possible. Use caution not to contaminate the coelomic cavity with yolk. After yolk sac removal, the opening into the coelomic cavity needs to be closed. Musculature and skin should be sutured closed and shells should have a protective sealing patch placed. If the yolk is hardened, is discolored, or has odor or if infection is suspected, culture and sensitivity of the yolk should be performed along with initiation of antimicrobial therapy.

Ill juveniles with a palpable mass in the abdomen, especially near the "umbilical" area visible on the skin, should be considered for exploratory surgery. If an abnormal yolk sac is identified, it can be surgically removed as listed above, followed by culture and sensitivity of the yolk and appropriate antimicrobial therapy.

Bone Diseases

Many different etiologies exist for bone diseases. Clinical signs of bone diseases include weakness, lameness, pathologic fractures, swelling of the bones, and visible skeletal deformities (scoliosis, kyphosis, and irregular carapace and plastron conformation in chelonia). Although bone diseases can occur in both juveniles and adults, the effects of bone diseases are often more clinically apparent and severe in juveniles afflicted during skeletal growth and development. A variety of conditions including osteomyelitis, osteitis, neoplasia, and an assortment of metabolic bone diseases can lead to bone disorders in reptiles and amphibians. A comprehensive review of the causes of and physiology of these diseases can be found in several reptile medicine texts.[4,5]

Calcium deficiency secondary to insufficient levels of dietary intake is often one of the first things many practitioners think of when seeing a patient with suspected metabolic bone disease. However, dietary calcium is only one component of metabolic bone diseases. A basic understanding of bone development and resorption, calcium physiology, and vitamin D_3 synthesis is important to fully assess and correct problems occurring. Inappropriate diets with mineral and vitamin deficiencies or excess should be assessed. If dietary calcium appears adequate and excessive phosphorous intake is not present, one must assess why the patient is experiencing calcium deficiency. Gastrointestinal disease can impair calcium and vitamin absorption, insufficient access to UVB lighting can impair vitamin D_3 synthesis, and inadequate vitamin D_3 can impair intestinal calcium absorption. Renal diseases can impair normal calcium and vitamin D physiology. Inability to properly regulate skin temperature, inadequate ability to exercise, or lack of production of certain hormones can also lead to skeletal malformations.

Vitamins A and D are important for normal development of bone and other tissues of the body. Some species obtain and successfully process oral sources of vitamin D to its active D_3 form. Most species require a variable amount of UVB radiation skin exposure and ability to obtain proper skin temperatures to allow the conversion of precursors of vitamin D_3 to its active form in many reptiles. There are significant differences between species and their requirements. Most reptiles and amphibians, with the exception of snakes and most monitors, require UVB light supplementation for normal bone development. Oversupplementation of vitamin D_3 and calcium can lead to metastatic mineralization and potentially other health problems.

Juvenile reptiles and amphibians with clinical signs of bone diseases should have a blood chemistry, including calcium and phosphorous, checked when possible. Plasma calcium levels may be normal in some cases where calcium is being mobilized away from the bones. Radiographs can often help differentiate causes of bone diseases. Characterization of lesions and subjective assessments of bone density can be made. Correction of diet and husbandry will often resolve mild conditions. Daily oral supplementation with calcium glubionate (23 mg/kg po q 24 h) and vitamin D_3 (OTC multivitamin powder supplements for reptiles) for 2 to 4 weeks during initial recovery often speeds recovery. Initial treatment with calcium gluconate injection(s) (50–100 mg/kg intracoelomic) should be considered for patients with severe hypocalcemia, profound weakness, and GI disease–induced problems. Calcium injections should not be continued long term. Analgesics should be used when bone pathology suggests a painful process. Culture and sensitivity of suspected osteomyelitis lesions or blood cultures are recommended followed by a minimum of 6 weeks of appropriate antimicrobial therapy. Some cases may take months to resolve and others may never resolve.

Shell Pyramiding

Abnormal development of the carapace in which the scutes are raised in the center, called "pyramiding," is common in captive raised tortoises. In the past the condition was thought to be related to improper diet. Research in *Geochelone sulcata* suggests that this abnormal shell development is primarily caused by insufficient environmental humidity.[6] Most juvenile tortoises spend much of their time in their burrow(s) in the wild. Burrow humidity is much higher than ground surface humidity even in arid environments. In captivity, where juvenile tortoises are housed indoors, the cage humidity is often lower that in their natural environments due to dry air from air conditioning and heating in houses. Cage humidity is often decreased further by supplemental heating sources in or on the enclosure.

Shell pyramiding is much more apparent in rapidly growing juveniles. Mild to moderate pyramiding does not appear to cause any significant long-term health concerns for tortoises. Severe pyramiding can lead to kyphosis and scoliosis, malposition of the pelvis, and subsequent problems walking correctly on the hind legs. When husbandry is corrected, pyramiding will often cease and normal smooth shell growth will occur at the scute margins.

Artificial burrow/shelter humidity can be increased in 1 of 2 ways. The substrate in the burrow/shelter can be slightly dampened as needed or a wooden burrow/shelter can be soaked in water as needed, both allowing for evaporative increase in the burrow/shelter humidity. If the environment is made too wet, there is an increased risk for skin, shell, and respiratory infections.

Predation and Cannibalism

Predation of juvenile reptiles and amphibians in the wild is common. Predators include many vertebrates and invertebrates. Predation in captivity can also occur. Other pets in or around the home such as dogs and cats and common insects such as ants and flies can attack juveniles, causing significant morbidity and mortality. Mice, crickets, and other live food items left in the cage for prolonged periods of time may also prey on small reptiles. Care should be taken to construct enclosures to prevent harm from predation.

Cannibalism can occur in many reptile species. This may either be by an adult or other larger sibling. In species such as bearded dragons, it is common for juveniles to bite off the toes and tails of others when group housed together. In general, juveniles of carnivorous and insectivorous reptiles should not be housed with larger conspecifics.

Gastrointestinal Foreign Bodies

Substrate selection needs to be made based on maintaining the proper environment for the species and minimization of ingestion. In smaller species, GI impactions may occur from ingestion of substrate larger than the intestinal lumen or large quantities of smaller substrate. Gravel, sand, bark and wood chips, ground walnut shell, fibrous plant materials, and any plastic or synthetic materials can cause GI obstructions. Food items such as prekilled mice or insects and damp or wet produce should be provided in ways that prevent cage substrate from adhering to them and being accidentally ingested. Small, colorful aquarium gravel may be ingested by chelonians and should not be used for them. Artificial plants should not be used in omnivorous and herbivorous reptile environments.

Anorexia and lethargy are the most common signs of GI foreign bodies. Diagnosis is usually made by coelomic palpation or radiographs. Administration of barium may be helpful in making a diagnosis, but many reptiles have very slow GI transit times compared to mammals and completion of a barium series may take days to weeks to complete. Intestinal foreign bodies can be managed medically or surgically. Both options carry different risks.

Medical management with rehydration and administration of lubricants and food may allow passage of some foreign bodies. There is risk of complete obstruction, severe intestinal dilation, and intestinal perforation. Surgery to remove impactions and foreign bodies may be challenging for smaller patients. Small suture and careful tissue handling must be used to prevent stricture.

Infectious Diseases and Parasitism

Many captive produced and wild caught reptiles and amphibians are exposed to an assortment of bacteria, viruses, parasites, and fungi that can cause disease as they go though the pet trade. They may be exposed to parasites and pathogens common to their species and others that are not. Large-scale production, shipping stress, multiple different holding environments, and other factors causing immunosuppression increase the morbidity and mortality from these parasites and pathogens. Ill juveniles should be worked up for diseases common to their species and diseases common to the pet trade in general.

Internal and external parasitism can create significant health problems for juvenile reptiles. Intestinal parasitism can cause diarrhea, GI gas, decreased appetite, and poor body condition and predispose to many other health problems. Often only small amounts of feces are available for examination. Desiccation and both hot and cold temperatures can have significant rapid negative effects on the samples diagnostic quality. For small reptiles, it is often best to use a combination of swabbing the cloaca with a moistened cotton swab and gentle caudal coelomic cavity massage and pressure to collect a diagnostic fecal sample. Sample sizes of 0.01 mL or even the mucus on the outside of the swab can be diagnostic with direct microscopic evaluation. One needs to look closely for areas containing bacteria and other cloacal components and evaluate parasite numbers in these areas. Finding 100 non-*Hexamita* flagellated protozoans dispersed through a slide can be insignificant. Finding 20 flagellated protozoans in one field of view or finding 1 *Hexamita* on a slide may identify a problem. In-house direct fecal examination should be performed on all reptile fecal samples. Samples sent to outside labs for flotation will only identify a small portion of parasitism problems.

Many flagellated protozoan parasites are present in reptiles. Some are pathogenic and others are not. Often, nonpathogenic protozoa are present in small numbers and no visible signs of disease are associated. Microscopic identification of 5 to 10 or more flagellated protozoans per ×40 power magnification of a direct fecal examination is enough to warrant treatment with metronidazole or ronidazole. Identification of coccidian parasites in the presence of disease warrants treatment with ponazuril. Most ciliated protozoa are not pathogenic and do not warrant treatment unless disease is present. An assortment of nematode parasites infect reptiles. Oxyurids are generally thought to be nonpathogenic in herbivorous reptiles and do not require treatment. Other nematodes present should be treated with drugs such as fenbendazole or pyrantel. Cestodes and trematodes can be treated with praziquantel; however, when encysted under the skin or internally, physical removal of the parasites is the only effective treatment.

Fecal cytology can also be a useful diagnostic tool. Identification of white blood cells and excessive amounts of a single bacterial type can be suggestive of bacterial enteritis. If bacterial enteritis is suspected, fecal culture is recommended.

Diseases affecting reptiles are too numerous to discuss here in depth. **Table 1** lists common diseases seen in juveniles and tests that can be performed with small sample sizes.

Table 1
Common problems in common pediatric patients and recommended diagnostics

	Clinical Signs	Common Causes	Initial Diagnostic Tests
Leopard gecko	Thin/underweight/skinny tails, diarrhea, anorexia	*Cryptosporidium*; intestinal parasites; bacterial enteritis Improper diet and husbandry	Direct microscopic exam of fresh feces. Fecal acid-fast staining or *Crytosporidium saurophilum* PCR
Bearded dragon	Thin/underweight, failure to grow, diarrhea, anorexia, lethargy, neurologic disease	Atadenovirus, intestinal parasites, bacterial enteritis Improper diet and husbandry	Direct (±floatation) microscopic exam of fresh feces. Fecal Atadenovirus PCR
Snakes (most species)	Thin/underweight, anorexia, intestinal gas, gastric swelling	Intestinal parasites, bacterial enteritis, *Cryptosporidium*	Fecal examination Gastric lavage for *Cryptosporidium serpentis* PCR
Lizards (most species)	Yellow crusting and/or ulcerative dermatitis	CANV, other fungal or bacterial dermatitis	Impression cytology. CANV PCR
Turtles and tortoises (most species)	Anorexia/hyporexia, diarrhea, failure to grow	Intestinal parasites, bacterial enteritis Improper diet and husbandry	Direct (±floatation) microscopic exam of fresh feces
Tortoises (most species)	Conjunctivitis, nasal and/or ocular discharge, inflamed choana	Mycoplasmosis or other bacterial upper respiratory infection	*Mycoplasma agassizii and testudinis* PCR; nasal lavage cytology
Amphibians (most species)	Lethargy, weight loss, anorexia/hyporexia, dermatitis	Viral, fungal, bacterial, and parasitic diseases	Direct microscopic exam of fresh feces, Ranavirus PCR, Chytrid PCR, impression cytology, cultures, water quality

Abbreviation: CANV, *Chrysosporium* anamorph of *Nannizziopsis vresii.*

HOSPITALIZATION AND PATIENT CARE

Hospitalization of juvenile reptiles and amphibians needs to take into account proper husbandry, thermoregulation, hydration, and nutritional support to allow proper recovery. Items used in the cages need to be washable and able to be disinfected or disposable. Deli cups or plastic bowls turned upside down with an entrance cut in one side can be used for shelters. Moistened paper towels can be placed in the hiding area. Plastic egg crating can be cut to necessary sizes and placed at an angle in the cage to allow climbing and basking. Overhead lighting and under the tank heating can be applied to one side of the enclosure.

Assist feeding is important for anorexic and hyporexic patients. Patients can be assist-fed their regular diet—prekilled small reptiles or rodents for carnivorous species, prekilled insects for insectivorous species, and small pieces of appropriate plant material for herbivorous reptiles. Lizards and chelonians will often swallow food items placed in their mouths. Snakes often need to have food items gently passed carefully into the caudal oral cavity or esophagus or they will regurgitate them. Several commercial syringe feeding diets are available such as Critical Care Fine Grind (Oxbow Animal Health, Murdock, NE, USA) and Emeraid products (Lafeber, Cornell, IL, USA). Many other mammalian diets have been used in reptiles with varying success. The physical characteristics and nutritional content of these diets may not match the natural or normal diet of some patients and can induce maldigestion and further GI problems. Make sure the product used has fiber, fat, and protein contents not too dissimilar to normal dietary requirements. Care needs to be taken not to overfeed patients with ileus and GI stasis, worsening these conditions. In general, 5 to 10 mL of food/kg can be given every 12 to 48 hours. Start with smaller, less frequent amounts and gradually increase based on patient response.

Rehydration and maintenance of proper hydration can be accomplished in several ways. For mildly dehydrated patients and to maintain proper hydration, oral and cloacal intake of fluids while soaking in a shallow water bath is often effective. As a general rule, the water bath should only come up to the ventral aspect of the chin of the reptile at rest to prevent drowning. Water temperature should be within the same temperature range as the environment it is kept in. For more debilitated reptiles, injectable fluids at a rate of 10 to 30 mL/kg per day are indicated for rehydration. Intravascular and intraosseous administration routes should be initially used on severely debilitated reptiles. Epicoelomic administration of fluids is preferred for chelonians. Subcutaneous and intracoelomic administration routes are preferred for geckos, lizards, monitors, and snakes. Electrolyte baths are often effective for amphibians.[7]

Medications

Medicating small neonatal and juvenile reptiles can be challenging. Caution must be used to prevent trauma to the jaw, oral cavity, or body overall when administrating oral medications. Intramuscular injection of medications that can cause damage to developing muscles should be avoided when possible.

Some medications have been linked to developmental problems. Fluoroquinolone antibiotics have been associated with numerous side effects in both juvenile and adult mammals. Although these side effects have not been documented in reptiles and amphibians, their use in juveniles should be avoided unless no other reasonable treatment options are available.

Oral medications may need to be compounded to lower concentrations for appropriate dosing of small patients. This can be performed by a compounding pharmacy or in the hospital by compounding prescriptions from tablets, capsules, or bulk powder. Consultation with a pharmacist is recommended if you are unfamiliar with proper compounding techniques and drug stability times. Premade suspensions can often be diluted with water to ease accurate dosing. Injectable medications may be indicated when oral administration is not possible. Injectable medications can often be diluted with sterile water for injection to dose appropriately.

Anesthesia and Surgery

Anesthesia and surgery are not commonly performed in herpetological pediatrics. Wound treatments and amputations are the most common procedures. Anesthesia and analgesia in juveniles can be accomplished with both inhalant and injectable medications. MS 222 and clove oil baths can be used to anesthetize amphibians. Care must be taken in calculating doses and administering anesthetics and analgesics in order to not overdose the patient. Intravenous catheters, with needles removed, can be used as endotracheal tubes for administration of inhalation anesthetics. Catheters can often be connected to small endotracheal tube connectors. Anesthetic monitoring can be performed via direct visualization of body changes associated with inflation/deflation of lungs, Doppler transducers positioned to listen to the heart rate, and, subjectively, the quality of the beat. Care must be taken to properly warm but not overheat smaller patients. A thermometer should be placed adjacent to the reptile to get an approximation of the patient's temperature.

Smaller surgical instruments made specifically for small patients, or vascular and ophthalmic surgical instruments are often necessary for proper tissue handling. Suture sizes of 5-0 and 6-0 may be necessary for closure of GI incisions in small patients. Sterile small gauze pads and micro cotton-tipped applicators are beneficial in surgery. Clear thin plastic drapes are also often beneficial for being able to visualize the patient during surgery.

Fracture management follows the same principles as with most larger vertebrates. External coaptation is often successful when the joints above and below the fracture are immobilized for 3–6 weeks. Limb fractures of lizards can often be managed by splinting the limb with applicator sticks or metal from paper clips molded into the correct position. Splinted front legs can be taped to the side of the body and hind legs taped to the tail. Spinal injuries resulting from trauma or pathology can often be managed by splinting and immobilizing the affected area when neurological function to the hind legs has not been lost. Amputation may be necessary for nonfixable fractures, necrotic limbs or digits, and other lesions.

Radiosurgery and CO_2 lasers decrease blood loss associated with surgical procedures. Caution needs to be taken to not create significant collateral tissue damage when using either of these surgical tools. Endoscopy can be used to allow gonad visualization for sex determination and coelomic cavity evaluation in large enough patients.

SUMMARY

Herpetological medicine and surgery requires knowledge and understanding of many different species. Herpetological pediatrics requires even more knowledge and understanding of the differences between adult and neonate, juvenile, and subadult patients. Proper environmental conditions and diet are critical to the health of growing reptiles, and providing the proper conditions and care for hospitalized patients is a vital component of treatment. Challenges often exist due to patient size. Exams, diagnostics, treatments, and surgeries can all be performed successfully on most pediatric patients. Flexibility in thought processes and techniques, the ability to adjust to the specific needs of each case, and some special small or fine equipment enable veterinarians to provide high-quality veterinary care to pediatric patients.

REFERENCES

1. Hernandez-Divers SJ, Stahl S, Farrell R. An endoscopic method for identifying sex of hatchling Chinese box turtles and comparison of general versus local anesthesia for laparoscopy. J Am Vet Med Assoc 2009;234:800–4.
2. Divers SJ. An introduction to reptile endoscopy. Proceedings of the Association of Reptilian and Amphibian Veterinarians. Kansas City (MO); 1998. p. 41–45.
3. Oftedal OT, Allen ME, Christopher TE. Dietary potassium affects food choice, nitrogen retention, and growth of desert tortoises. Proceedings of the Desert Tortoise Council Symposium. 1995. p. 58–61.
4. Calvert I. Nutritional problems. In: Girling S, Raiti P, editors. BSAVA manual of reptiles. 2nd edition. Gloucester (UK): BSAVA; 2004. p. 289–308.
5. Mader DR. Metabolic bone diseases. In: Mader DR, editor. Reptile medicine and surgery. 2nd edition. St Louis (MO): Saunders; 2006. p. 841–51.
6. Weisner CS, Iben C. Influence of environmental humidity and dietary protein on the pyramidal growth of carapaces of African spurred tortoises, Geochelone sulcata. J Anim Physiol Anim Nutr 2003;87:66–74.
7. Wright KM, Whitaker BR. Pharmacotherapeutics. In: Wright KM, Whitaker BR, editors. Amphibian medicine and captive husbandry. Malabar (FL): Krieger Publishing; 2001. p. 309–30.

Approaches to Management and Care of the Neonatal Nondomestic Ruminant

Barbara A. Wolfe, DVM, PhD, Dipl. ACZM[a],*, Nadine Lamberski, DVM, Dipl. ACZM[b]

KEYWORDS

• Neonate • Pediatric • Antelope • Deer • Ungulate

Veterinary care of the newborn nondomestic ruminant can be both rewarding and very challenging, with some practitioners reporting high mortality rates before 6 months of age.[1] Case management during the critical neonatal period is typically modeled after management of domestic ruminants; however, some unique differences exist between nondomestic ungulates and their domestic counterparts that affect neonatal management and medical care. These differences become apparent quickly when the nondomestic neonate requires treatment, and an understanding of the special needs and risks involved can prevent unnecessary problems and losses. The aim of this article is to discuss the unique challenges presented by nondomestic ruminants and approaches to management of neonatal and pediatric cases.

MANAGING THE DAM

Preparation for neonatal and pediatric care should begin when the dam is known to be pregnant. In nondomestic ruminants, early diagnosis of pregnancy is uncommon due to the increased manipulation and stress associated with handling for rectal palpation or ultrasound. For many species, fecal progestin assays have been developed, providing a means of noninvasive pregnancy diagnosis.[2–5] However, this procedure often requires time-intensive repeated fecal collection from the dam (generally 2–5 samples per week) for the duration of 1 estrous cycle plus 2 or more weeks to verify maintenance of elevated progesterone. Several zoological institutions have endocrinology laboratories that may provide endocrine assessments as a service. Rectal palpation and ultrasound examination should be conducted opportunistically, such as for annual examination, hoof

The authors have nothing to disclose.

[a] Department of Animal Health, Columbus Zoo and Aquarium and the Wilds, 9900 Riverside Drive, Columbus, OH 43065, USA

[b] Veterinary Clinical Operations, San Diego Zoo Safari Park, 15500 San Pasqual Valley Road, Escondido, CA 92027, USA

* Corresponding author.

E-mail address: bwolfe@thewilds.org

work, or other medical care, for females suspected to be pregnant. However, the risk of anesthesia may outweigh the benefit of early pregnancy diagnosis in many fractious species. Stillbirths are not uncommon in nondomestic ruminants anesthetized repeatedly during pregnancy.

Preparation for successful birth and mother-rearing should emphasize health and reduced disturbance to the dam. If possible, fractious nondomestic ruminants should give birth in an environment to which they are accustomed. Inexperienced dams, particularly those that have not observed maternal behavior in a herd setting, should be monitored closely near parturition. Species with strong herd instincts may be most successful when housed with conspecifics during calving season, and many will demonstrate birth synchrony.[6,7] However, wild ruminant species vary widely in social grouping and behavior, and captive grouping can affect reproductive success.[8] Research into the best captive social environment for the species in question before birth can maximize the chance of successful birth and maternal care. Timing exposure of females to males in nonseasonal or seasonally polyestrous species to maximize the chance of late spring or early summer births in temperate zones can also improve neonatal survival in pasture-managed animals. Housing should provide the opportunity for seclusion, adequate ventilation and drainage, and exposure to sunlight to reduce pathogen levels.

Vaccination of dams for diseases of regional risk approximately 2 months before expected parturition can optimize levels of specific immunoglobulins (Igs) in colostrum and improve neonatal health. Vaccination at this time for diseases of particular concern to neonates such as *Clostridium* sp, *Escherichia coli*, rotavirus, coronavirus, and bovine viral diarrhea is common practice in domestic ruminants.[9–11] However, live vaccines should be used with caution in nondomestic ruminants. One month before expected birth, the energy ration should be increased and special attention paid to the provision of adequate calcium and minerals, particularly if the regional soil is deficient in specific minerals, such as selenium.

General signs of impending parturition include teat and udder enlargement, which can occur days to weeks before birth depending on the species, and vulvar swelling/relaxation. Vulvar changes generally occur closer to parturition than udder enlargement. Dams will often seek isolation just before birth and will often give birth to live offspring at night, while stillbirths and abortions can occur at any time.

PREPARATION FOR BIRTH

While most ruminants are capable of successfully delivering and raising offspring, nondomestic ungulates in zoos and related institutions are often housed in unnatural social or environmental situations, increasing the chances of dystocia, conspecific trauma, and maternal neglect. If a neonate requires medical care, it may be impractical to house the animal with its dam due to the need for frequent separation, stress on the dam, and the likelihood of maternal rejection. Therefore, preparations for neonatal care should include a hand-rearing protocol, which should detail record keeping, equipment/supplies, formula and supplements needed, housing, and socialization. The Association of Zoos and Aquariums' Nutrition Advisory Group (http://www.nagonline.net/) and the book, *Hand-Rearing Wild and Domestic Animals,*[12] are practical hand-rearing resources. Veterinary preparations include plans for treatment of failure of passive transfer (FPT, discussed later). Plans to acquire plasma, colostrum, and milk replacer formulas should be in place before birth.

BIRTH AND POSTPARTUM CARE
Dystocia
Identification of dystocia requiring intervention can be complicated in nondomestic ruminants. While anterior dorsosacral presentation of the fetus with forelimbs extended is by far the most common, posterior dorsosacral presentation with the hindlimbs extended is very common in some species, such as Pere David's deer (*Elaphurus davidianus*) and red deer (*Cervus elaphus*) and may or may not cause difficulty in parturition. The most common causes of dystocia in cattle are malpresentation of the fetus and maternofetal disproportion. Dystocia is not uncommon in nondomestic ruminants, particularly in species of limited genetic diversity, and represents an important risk factor for morbidity and mortality in domestic[13] and nondomestic calves. In fact, beef calves born following dystocia are 2 to 6 times more likely than normal-birth calves to develop disease within 45 days of birth.[14,15] Nondomestic ruminant neonates are at even greater risk than domestic calves following dystocia due to the necessity of general anesthesia for birth intervention. Furthermore, many dams will not accept an offspring following general anesthesia, resulting in FPT and the need for hand-rearing. Hypoxemia and acidosis in the calf (discussed later) are possible sequelae to dystocia that may also lead to FPT, although it is unclear whether this is due to a direct effect on Ig absorption or to resulting weakness and inability of the neonate to stand and nurse.[16]

NEONATAL TRIAGE AND TREATMENT
The Decision to Treat
In beef cattle, 69% of calf losses before weaning occur within 96 hours of birth,[17] underscoring the need for early intervention. While early intervention is also critical in nondomestic ruminants, the decision to treat can be more involved than in domestic operations.

Maternal neglect is a common occurrence resulting in the need for neonatal care in nondomestic ruminants. Dams that are inexperienced, ill, housed in unnatural social or environmental situations, or stressed by human presence are the most likely to reject a neonate. However, the practitioner must keep in mind during the decision-making process that when an experienced dam abandons her offspring, it may be due to a congenital, infectious, or metabolic problem compromising its viability. In such cases, a significant amount of money and time can be put into a neonate whose survival is unlikely.

If treatment requires that the dam and offspring be brought into confinement, the dam may become inappetant, reject the neonate, or both. In some species, such as sable antelope (*Hippotragus niger*), reintroduction of the dam back into the herd following isolation with her calf can be problematic, leading to conspecific aggression and injury.

In many species, the sex of the neonate is a significant factor in the decision to treat. Hand-raised animals will usually demonstrate altered social behaviors as adults, including an inappropriate response to humans. Male ruminants that are hand-reared may thereby pose an intolerable risk as adults in captivity by demonstrating a lack of fear and increased aggression toward humans. Alternatively, hand-reared females may provide a benefit to the herd by showing less aversion to human presence than their herdmates. Such females are useful in "calming" the herd during intensive management, as companions to conspecifics requiring hospitalization, or as surrogate dams to hand-reared neonates, easing the transition of the neonate into the herd. Strategies for socialization of hand-reared neonates are discussed later. The monetary and labor costs of committing to treatment and hand-rearing, the risk to the dam, the likelihood of success, and the future of the neonate must all be taken into account in the decision to treat a compromised newborn nondomestic ruminant.

Critical Care of the Postpartum Neonate

Neonates born following dystocia or under extreme environmental conditions are more likely to require resuscitation and medical care than those experiencing normal birth conditions. Once the decision is made to treat these cases, early intervention is essential. Dystocia is likely to cause both respiratory and metabolic acidosis. Following normal birth, mild respiratory acidosis may occur for a few hours and metabolic acidosis for up to 48 hours.[18] However, severe acidosis can result in reduced vigor, decreased suckling response and an increased chance of FPT.[19] A good indicator of acidosis is time to sternal recumbency: in cattle, more than 15 minutes to sternal recumbency is associated with low survival.[20] Poor muscle tone and decreased pedal reflexes are also suggestive of acidosis. Scleral and conjunctival hemorrhage indicate both hypoxia and acidosis and can also signal a poor prognosis.[21]

Establishment of a patent airway, initiation of a normal breathing pattern, and establishing adequate circulation are the first priorities in the treatment of a critical neonate. In general, cardiac resuscitation is not indicated, as neonates born without a heart beat are not likely to survive.[15] Attention should be paid to physical stimulation of the neonate, as severe acidosis may cause depression of the central reflexes that initiate respiration.[15] To clear the airway, place the neonate in sternal recumbency and clear fluids and physical obstructions by hand or suction. Rub the neonate vigorously with towels or bedding to simulate the phrenic nerve, which innervates the diaphragm. If respiration is not immediately initiated, stimulation of the nasal passage or pharynx with a finger or piece of straw should induce an inspiratory reflex. Acupuncture at the philtrum may also stimulate respiration.[22]

Neonates born to anesthetized dams may have respiratory depression resulting from pharmacologic sedation, and specific antagonists should be administered to the neonate as well as to the dam. Doxapram hydrochloride stimulates central chemoreceptors and may be beneficial in calves born with mild respiratory suppression, but it is unlikely to be effective in severely depressed neonates. Use of doxapram as a respiratory stimulant has demonstrated varying results,[23–25] but it may improve acid-base balance.[22] If these methods are unsuccessful, endotracheal intubation and positive pressure ventilation are preferable to mouth-to-nose ventilation for providing respiratory support. Oxygen therapy, if available, has been shown to improve neonatal survival in at-risk domestic calves and is best administered via endotracheal tube.[15]

Placement of an intravenous catheter and fluid therapy as necessary can improve the chance of survival in compromised neonates, and provides a means of treating metabolic abnormalities rapidly. Metabolic acidosis can be treated with a bolus of sodium bicarbonate (1–2 mEq/kg)[19] *following* the establishment of a normal breathing pattern. Treatment before establishing normal breathing, however, is likely to exacerbate respiratory acidosis.

Maintenance of appropriate body temperature is easily overlooked during resuscitation and care of the neonate but essential to its survival, particularly in critical cases that fail to demonstrate normal thermoregulatory mechanisms such as shivering. In domestic calves, provision of an external heat source for 24 hours postpartum has been shown to improve not only body temperature but also oxygen saturation, tidal volume, and respiratory rate.[26]

IDENTIFYING ILLNESS IN YOUNG RUMINANTS

Despite apparently normal birth, behavior and maternal care, illness is not uncommon in nondomestic ruminants under 30 days of age. Most mortality in domestic calves following a normal birth is due to prematurity, congenital defects, or infection.[15] Close observation of neonates soon after birth is important to document normal behavior and suckling, but an understanding of species-specific behavior is necessary. While domestic calves are precocial "followers" and stand and follow the dam soon after birth, 75% of nondomestic ruminants are characterized as "hiders.[6]" These neonates are left by their mothers to lie motionless, reunited only for infrequent nursing periods for the first days to months, depending on the species. In these species, failure to observe the neonate nursing, or to find it, may lead the inexperienced observer to assume the neonate is ill. Hippotragine antelopes and deer are frequently "hider" neonates, whereas wild cattle, goat-like species, and gazelles are usually "followers." Neonates should be observed nursing within a few hours of birth. Observation of a calf that is weak or unresponsive to stimulation by the dam, demonstrates prolonged unsuccessful or no attempts to nurse, or is too weak to stand soon after birth indicates a need for evaluation.

Approach to Illness in Neonatal and Young Ruminants

Common causes of illness in neonatal ruminants include acidosis, hypothermia, hypoglycemia, dehydration, pneumonia, and septicemia.[10,15] Each of these conditions can progress rapidly to death, and often more than one is present in the sick neonate,[27] necessitating expeditious diagnosis and treatment of existing conditions. **Table 1** describes the diagnosis and treatment of common conditions in the sick neonatal ruminant.

Bacterial septicemia is common in compromised neonatal ruminants, primarily due to inadequate colostral intake and establishment of immunocompetence. In the neonate, the primary source of bacterial contamination of blood is the intestine due to nonspecific pinocytosis. In older calves, enteritis may cause septicemia through loss of integrity of the intestinal wall. By the second or third week of age, omphalophlebitis, arthritis, pneumonia, and meningitis may result in septicemia.[28] Septicemic calves between 2 and 6 days of age present with vague signs such as altered mentation (ranging from mild signs to coma), depression, or decreased suckle response with or without diarrhea. The condition is most often rapidly fatal. Physical exam findings may include hypothermia or hyperthermia, tachycardia, tachypnea, hyperemia or petechiae of mucous membranes, increased capillary refill time, cold extremities, and diminished peripheral pulse. Point-of-care testing is likely to reveal hypoglycemia, metabolic acidosis, hypoxia, and hypotension. Observation of any combination of these signs should lead the practitioner to suspect septicemia and/or meningitis and act quickly. Blood culture before initiation of antibiotics is prudent. Treatment should include fluid therapy and intravenous antibiotics, the choice of which should include activity against both gram-negative and gram-positive bacteria. Commonly encountered pathogens and resistance patterns at the institution should also be considered when choosing antibiotics. Nonsteroidal anti-inflammatory drugs are helpful in modulating the inflammatory response once hydration is corrected. Correction of hypothermia and hypoglycemia should be addressed immediately (see **Table 1**). When treating a hypoglycemic neonate, dextrose may be delivered intraperitoneally if venous access is a challenge due to profound hypotension or dehydration. Check blood glucose frequently during the initial 24 hours of treatment. Inability to correct hypoglycemia despite treatment is suggestive of septicemia.

Table 1 Approach to diagnosis and treatment of common conditions in the sick neonate		
Condition	Diagnosis	Treatment
Hypothermia	94–99°F (34.4–37°C) = hypothermia Below 94°F = severe hypothermia	Warm neonate slowly (2°F per hour) using dry circulating air, blankets, heat lamps and administration of warmed IV fluids or warmed oral colostrum.
Hypoglycemia	Blood glucose <60 mg/dL	Deliver 500 mg/kg (10 mL/kg 5% solution) dextrose IV over several minutes. Repeated dosing may be necessary to increase blood glucose to an acceptable level. Once corrected, maintain glucose administration at least 250 mg/kg/day until neonate accepts food, or begin parenteral nutrition.
Metabolic acidosis	Base deficit >10 mmol/L Blood pH <7.25	Intravenous sodium bicarbonate (1.3%): • mEq HCO_3 = Base deficit x body wt x 0.5. • Empirical treatment with 1–2 mEq/kg
Hypoxemia	SaO_2 <90% PaO_2 <70 mmHg	Nasal insufflation with O_2 5–10 L/h or ventilation
Septicemia	a. Blood culture positive for bacterial pathogens b. Elevated or reduced white blood cell count c. Fibrinogen >500 mg/dL d. >2% band neutrophils	Initiate broad spectrum intravenous antibiotics; consider plasma transfusion; monitor and correct aberrations in body temperature, hydration, acid/base balance, and blood glucose; provide adequate nutrition.

Supportive treatment for neonatal septicemia should include provision of a clean, warm, lowly lit environment; soft, clean bedding; intravenous fluid supplementation; and plasma transfusion, colostrum supplementation, or milk-based nutritional support, depending on the age of the neonate. Bedding should be changed frequently as septicemic neonates are usually too weak to stand and therefore susceptible to urine scald and corneal irritation/ulceration. If the patient is normothermic (≥98°F) and responsive, offer a bottle as soon as it appears strong enough to suckle.

Assessing Passive Transfer

Maternal immunity is not transferred in utero in ruminants. Therefore, neonatal ruminants rely on the intestinal absorption of antibodies from colostrum, produced by the dam in the first 24 hours postpartum, for humoral protection from environmental pathogens. Endogenous production of antibodies by the calf does not reach protective levels until at least 1 month of age. While observation of a strong neonate suckling normally from the dam in the first hours after birth is a practical indicator of successful passive transfer, the performance of neonatal physical exams on all calves is a good practice. This exam allows the practitioner to check for medical and congenital conditions, apply an identification tag, supplement vitamin E and selenium if needed, and collect blood for passive transfer testing if maternal care is in question. Detection of IgG in plasma is possible as soon as 2 hours after a colostrum feeding. Therefore, timing of neonatal physical exams may be determined by many factors, such as the mobility

Table 2
Common tests for assessing passive transfer.

Passive Transfer Test	Description	Result Indicating FPT
Sodium Sulfite Turbidity Test	Sodium sulfite causes precipitation of antibodies. Mix 14%, 16% and 18% sodium sulfite. Add 0.1 ml serum to 1.9 mL of each concentration in separate tubes. Mix and observe at 1 hour. Commercially available as a kit; simple and quick; high sensitivity, low specificity[16]	Precipitation or flakes at all 3 concentrations 3+ = >1500 mg/dL. 2+ = 500–1500 mg/dl (partial FPT). 1+ = <500 mg/dL (FPT). 86% accurate in detecting FPT.[29]
Zinc Sulfate Turbidity Test	Similar to sodium sulfite test but more susceptible to error due to hemolysis. Add 0.1 ml serum to 6 ml of a 350 mg/mL $ZnSO_4$ solution. Cap, mix and observe turbidity at 1 hour.	Turbidity insufficient to obscure newsprint indicates FPT.[29]
Serum Total Protein	Simple refractometer test. TP may be affected by dehydration, leading to a false positive result.	<5.2–5.5 g/dL TP indicates FPT.[30]
Glutaraldehyde Coagulation Test	Relies on the induction of coagulation of antibodies by glutaraldehyde. Add 1 mL serum to 50 μL 10% glutaraldehyde and observe clot formation in 1 hour. High specificity, low sensitivity.	Complete clot = >600 mg/dL. Semisolid clot = 400–600 mg/dl. Failure to observe clot formation indicates FPT.[29,31]
Serum Gamma-Glutamyltransferase (GGT)	Serum levels of GGT are high following colostrum feeding. Relies on in-house serum testing ability or laboratory time. Best as an adjunct to other tests.	<50 IU/l in domestic calves indicates FPT.[16,30] Varies with species, but GGT levels <50X normal adult serum levels are suggestive of FPT.

of the neonate, the observation (or lack thereof) of nursing and the ability to find "hider" species in large pastures. Generally, the behavior of the dam of hider species is a very poor guide to the location of the neonate.

Common tests for passive transfer are listed in **Table 2**. While radial immunodiffusion is considered the gold standard test for passive transfer, it is a species-specific laboratory test and not practical for rapid diagnosis of FPT in nondomestic ruminants. Similarly, an enzyme-linked immunosorbent assay, while useful as a stall-side test for domestic calves, is also a species-specific test and therefore not practical for nondomestic species. Several commercially available tests, as described in **Table 2**, are sufficiently sensitive to rapidly identify FPT to allow for the immediate development of a treatment plan.

Treating Failure of Passive Transfer

In domestic calves, colostrum absorption occurs during the first 24 to 36 hours of life. The timing of this nonselective absorption of macromolecules including IgG ends approximately 24 hours after the first meal.[32] Peak Ig transfer across the enterocytes occurs during the first 4 hours postpartum and declines rapidly after 12 hours[33–35]; therefore early colostrum intake should result in higher IgG serum concentration. Peak serum IgG concentration occurs 32 hours postpartum.[15] FPT occurs when inadequate levels of IgG are absorbed, predisposing the neonate to the development of disease. Even calves nursing from their dams can experience FPT by ingesting an inadequate volume of colostrum during the critical time period or by ingesting colostrum of relatively low IgG content. FPT calves experience higher rates of neonatal mortality, and this higher mortality rate can extend to the postweaning period.[16]

The decision to treat a calf with FPT and the method of treatment should be based on several factors including the animal's age, species, value, and environment and the availability of colostrum, plasma, and other resources. Calves suffering from FPT are at greater risk for developing disease but can survive if placed in a clean environment with low exposure to infectious pathogens. Immunocompetent calves are able to produce approximately 1 g of IgG per day.[35,36] Despite this, they cannot respond to certain antigens, such as gram-negative bacteria, until 30 days of age.[37] The prophylactic use of broad-spectrum, parenteral antimicrobials in calves with FPT should be considered but must be combined with colostrum replacement and management practices that minimize pathogen exposure.[16]

FPT calves less than 24 hours of age can be treated orally with fresh colostrum, commercial colostrum replacer, or plasma. It is very difficult to collect a volume of colostrum sufficient to prevent FPT from a lactating nondomestic ruminant. Bovine colostrum is an alternative, but there is an inherent risk of disease transmission (eg, Johne disease) associated with this practice. Commercial colostrum replacers are therefore recommended for neonatal nondomestic ruminants. Serum contains significantly lower IgG concentrations than does colostrum and is thereby not a good choice for oral administration. Commercial hyperimmune plasma, however, is a viable alternative. Oral administration should be attempted first with a bottle, but weak calves or those that do not take readily to a bottle should receive colostrum via oroesophageal intubation (see below) or parenteral plasma transfusion.

During the first 24 hours of life, colostrum should be fed at a volume equal to 10% of the neonate's body weight divided over several feedings. Higher volumes should be fed (up to 15% body weight) if the source is poor quality colostrum or plasma. Ideally, as much colostrum as possible should be fed within the first 4 hours to maximize absorption of IgG. In domestic calves, 100 g colostral IgG delivered in the first feeding is associated with lower rates of FPT.[38] When using a colostrum replacer purchased as a powder, the actual IgG dose fed can be varied by mixing the powder with different volumes of water. However, while making a very concentrated formula may seem logical, this may not be palatable to the calf. A recent study in springbok (*Antidorcas marsupialis*) calves has shown that using a commercial bovine colostrum replacer at a dose of greater than 4.68 g/dL of IgG per kg of body weight divided into 5 feedings over 24 hours resulted in passive transfer rates that were comparable to calves consuming maternal colostrum (Lamberski, personal communication, 2011). Colostrum can still be administered orally beyond 24 hours of age, as intraluminal colostrum provides local protection.

When colostrum is not available, plasma can be administered orally or parenterally in calves less than 24 hours old, or parenterally after 24 hours of age. Plasma is typically administered at a rate of 20–40 mL/kg IV. Whole blood can be administered instead of plasma, but the volume should be increased to account for the presence of red blood cells. If plasma or whole blood is unavailable, the use of commercial plasma is an option. Commercially available equine plasma has been used successfully in nondomestic ruminants to prevent FPT.[39] Plasma can also be administered intraperitoneally (IP). This procedure is less invasive and intensive than IV administration and allows the calf to be returned to the dam in a shorter period of time. While the recommended plasma dose for intravenous administration is 40 ml/kg, IP administration may require a larger volume of plasma. To administer plasma IP, an area in the left paralumbar fossa is clipped and surgically prepared. A needle is inserted through the skin, abdominal musculature, and peritoneum in the center of the paralumbar fossa. Alternatively, local anesthesia can be used before making a stab incision and then inserting an 18 gauge × 2 inch over-the-needle indwelling catheter. Plasma can be delivered at a relatively rapid drip rate.[16] Calves should be monitored for adverse reactions (lethargy, fever, tachypnea, tachycardia) during parenteral plasma administration regardless of the route, and those receiving plasma from an animal anesthetized using opioid anesthetics may benefit from naltrexone administration during plasma administration.

Despite the method of treatment, tests for FPT should be repeated following treatment and the animal retreated if adequate passive transfer is not confirmed.

LONG-TERM CARE AND SOCIALIZATION
Nutrition

Neonatal ruminants requiring treatment are most often, as mentioned above, raised in the absence of their dam, necessitating hand-rearing. Even if a calf is allowed to remain with the dam, supplemental feeding may be necessary. In some cases, neonates can be returned to the natal group following a period of stabilization and training to ensure reliable consumption of formula from a bottle. This approach has the added benefits of optimal socialization and minimal staff time.

Milk composition is influenced by genetics, nutrition, and environmental factors, and the components vary substantially between species.[40] Therefore, it is not possible to recommend a hand-raising formula that is suitable for all nondomestic ruminant species. A formula's composition should mimic that of the dam's milk in protein, carbohydrate (lactose), fat, and total solids ratios. Many commercial milk replacers are available but the authors have experience with LAND O LAKES Doe's Match (Land O'Lakes Animal Milk Products, Shoreview, MN, USA)[a] and Zoologic Milk Matrix (PetAg, Inc., Hampshire, IL, USA).[b] Goat's milk is often used and is a good choice for many species, used alone or in combination with a milk replacer. However, unless fortified, goat's milk does not contain vitamin E and is relatively low in zinc and copper. Most milk is naturally low in iron. For these reasons, a vitamin and mineral supplement is often added to the formula. Adding probiotics to the formula may be beneficial in establishing a healthy rumen flora.

In the first 2 to 3 weeks of a ruminant's life, termed the preruminant phase, digestion of milk occurs in the abomasum and small intestine. During this phase, milk deposited into the nonfunctional rumenoreticulum (eg, via tube feeding) is not digested and often leads to rumenitis and septicemia.[41] Reflex closure of the esophageal groove, stimulated by suckling, normally prevents this deposition. If tube feeding is required during this time, the tube can be passed to the mid-esophagus to stimulate swallowing and closure of the groove. Additionally, milk feeding can be preceded by oral administration of 10% sodium bicarbonate or 2–5% copper sulfate, which facilitates groove closure for several minutes.[42] Esophageal feeding should be conducted using gravity flow.

---

[a]http://www.lolmilkreplacer.com/KID/DoesMatchMilkReplacer/default.aspx.
[b]http://www.petag.com/industry/zoologic-formulation-mixing/.

During the transitional phase, which begins at 2 to 3 weeks of age, the calf begins to take in small amounts of dry feed and the volatile fatty acids butyric and propionic acid stimulate differentiation of the ruminal papillae.[43] By this age, the neonate should be provided with a variety of appropriate hay, pelleted ration, and calf supplements to begin to sample, in addition to the milk ration. From initiation of solid feed through weaning, sand or dirt ingestion is common in some areas. Sand ingestion can be due to formula imbalances, gastrointestinal diseases, stress, or boredom, but determining the exact etiology is often difficult. Impaction can result as can the need for medical and/or surgical intervention. Since ingestion can lead to impaction, it is best recognized early as a symptom of an underlying problem. The calf should be housed away from sand or dirt while the etiologies are explored, and it may be necessary to attempt formula changes in lieu of a diagnosis as the exact imbalance may not be obvious. Early weaning may be considered in some cases.

Abnormal fecal consistency (liquid, loose, log-shaped, or clumped stool) is not uncommon during the first few months, particularly if the animal is being hand-reared. There are many etiologies for changes in fecal consistency, ranging from formula intolerance to enteritis, necessitating close monitoring of fecal output and consistency until weaning. The transition from preruminant to ruminant and the weaning process both result in changes in gastrointestinal flora and, often, fecal consistency. High-carbohydrate feeds or an overconsumption of carbohydrates can result in clostridial overgrowth and diarrhea. As in domestic ruminants, nondomestic ruminants may benefit from vaccination against *Clostridium perfringens* type C and D at 4 and 8 weeks of age.

The weaning process if often initiated at 2 months of age but is not complete until 3 to 4 months of age. This varies with species and health status and can be accelerated in the interest of returning the animal to its herd, or if formula intolerance is a concern. Conversely, the weaning process can be slowed considerably if an animal has difficulty accepting solid food.

Socialization

Ruminants that are hand-raised need to be socialized before introduction to their herd. If animals will remain in the collection, plans to reintroduce the animal to the herd should be in place by the end of the weaning period. It is ideal to hand-raise nondomestic ruminants with conspecifics or other nondomestic ruminants of similar age. Herd-adapted species need the psychological benefits that result from companionship. They also need a playmate to ensure adequate bouts of activity and exercise. If another hand-reared animal is not available, an older, calm "aunt" is a suitable substitute. Using an older animal has the added benefit of exposing the hand-reared animal to normal fecal flora. Before reintroduction to the herd, it is beneficial to first introduce it to a companion animal to reduce the chance of rejection by the herd. Once bonded, the pair can be introduced together. This is particularly valuable when the animal was raised with a species other than its own.

In some cases it is of benefit to raise young ruminants without imprinting them significantly on humans. For instance, hand-reared male elk and other species imprinted on humans can be very dangerous as adults. A plan to reduce imprinting should be in place within the first few days of life and continue until weaning and complete introduction to the herd. **Fig. 1** depicts a device for hand-rearing that minimizes exposure to human presence and scent. A framed box large enough for a person to stand in is covered with tarp or heavy cloth. The front of the box consists of a 2-way mirror and 2 hand-sized ports for feeding the calf. The handler

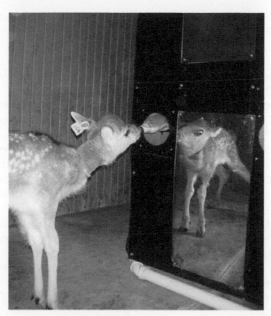

Fig. 1. An approach to hand-rearing that minimizes social imprinting on humans. The handler enters the box from the rear and views the neonate through a two-way mirror, feeding through ports in the front of the box.

enters the box from behind, avoiding being seen by the calf, and carries the box toward the calf. Alternatively, the calf can be trained with a clicker to approach the box. The handler uses leather gloves that may be covered with conspecific female urine to encourage appropriate scent recognition and feeds the neonate with a bottle using the ports in the front of the box, avoiding exposure of the arms. The 2-way mirror allows the handler to see the neonate, but the neonate sees itself. This type of device has been used in combination with early weaning and reintroduction to the herd to raise orphaned male ungulates to be socially normal herd members as adults.

SUMMARY

Management and care of the nondomestic ruminant neonate are similar in principle to domestic animal practice. Housing of the dam, conditions for birth, preparation for intervention, and plans for treatment and hand-rearing of sick neonates must all be considered carefully before undertaking nondomestic ruminant breeding. Unfortunately, neonatal losses tend to be much higher in nondomestic calves before weaning than in domestic cattle, sheep, and goat herds.[1] With continued habitat and population declines in wild species, successful captive breeding of nondomestic herds becomes more important to species sustainability and potential reintroduction programs. The primary challenges contributing to neonatal losses in nondomestic ruminants are often animal temperament and adaptation to captivity. Only through experience can some of these challenges be overcome. However, by understanding some species-specific behavioral tendencies and the fractious nature of nondomestic ruminants in general, we can improve our success in managing and maintaining healthy populations of nondomestic ruminants in captivity.

REFERENCES

1. Barnes R, Greene K, Holland J, et al. Management and husbandry of duikers at the Los Angeles Zoo. Zoo Biol 2002;21:107–21.
2. Brown JL, Wasser SK, Wildt DE, et al. Faecal steroid analysis for monitoring ovarian and testicular function in diverse mild carnivore, primate and ungulate species. Zeitschrift Fur Saugetierkunde 1997;62:27–31.
3. Graham L, Schwarzenberger F, Mostl E, et al. A versatile enzyme immunoassay for the determination of progestogens in feces and serum. Zoo Biol 2001;20:227–36.
4. Pickard AR, Abaigar T, Green DI, et al. Hormonal characterization of the reproductive cycle and pregnancy in the female Mohor gazelle (Gazella dama mhorr). Reproduction 2001;122:571–80.
5. del Castillo SM, Bashaw MJ, Patton ML, et al. Fecal steroid analysis of female giraffe (Giraffa camelopardalis) reproductive condition and the impact of endocrine status on daily time budgets. Gen Comp Endocrinol 2005;141:271–81.
6. Thompson KV. Spatial integration in infant sable antelope, Hippotragus niger. Anim Behav 1998;56:1005–14.
7. Ims RA. The ecology and evolution of reproductive synchrony. Trends Ecol Evol 1990;5:135–40.
8. Price EE, Stoinski TS. Group size: determinants in the wild and implications for the captive housing of wild mammals in zoos. Appl Anim Beh Sci 2007;103:255–64.
9. LeBlanc SJ, Lissemore KD, Kelton DF, et al. Major advances in disease prevention in dairy cattle. J Dairy Sci 2006;89:1267–79.
10. Menzies P. Lambing management and neonatal care. In: Youngquist RS, editor. Current therapy in large animal theriogenology. 2nd edition. St Louis (MO): Saunders Elsevier; 2007. p. 680–95.
11. Ellis JA, Hassard LE, Cortese VS, et al. Effects of perinatal vaccination on humoral and cellular immune responses in cows and young calves. J Am Vet Med Assoc 1996; 208:393–400.
12. Stringfield C, Greene K. Exotic ungulates. In: Gage L, editor. Hand-rearing wild and domestic mammals. Ames (IA): Iowa State Press; 2002. p. 256–62.
13. Laster DB, Gregory KE. Factors influencing perinatal and early postnatal calf mortality. J Anim Sci 1973;37:1092–7.
14. Toombs RE, Wikse SE, Kasari TR. The incidence, causes and financial impact of perinatal mortality in North American beef herds. Vet Clin N Am Food Anim Pract 1994;10:137–46.
15. Nagy DW. Resuscitation and critical care of neonatal calves. Vet Clin N Am Food Anim Pract 2009;25:1–12.
16. Weaver DM, Tyler JW, VanMetre DC, et al. Passive transfer of colostral immunoglobulins in calves. J Vet Intern Med 2000;14:569–77.
17. Bellows RA, Patterson DJ, Burfening PJ, et al. Occurrence of neonatal and postnatal mortality in range beef cattle. 2. Factors contributing to calf death. Theriogenology 1987;28:573–86.
18. Szenci O, Taverne MAM, Bakonyi S, et al. Comparison between prenatal and postnatal acid-base status of calves and their perinatal mortality. Vet Q 1988;10: 140–4.
19. Grove-White D. Resuscitation of the newborn calf. In Pract 2000;22:17.
20. Schuijt G, Taverne MAM. The interval between birth and sternal recumbency as an objective measure of the vitality of newborn calves. Vet Rec 1994;135:111–5.

21. Noakes DE, Parkinson TJ, England GCW, et al, editors. Arthur's veterinary reproduction and obstetrics. 8th edition. London/New York: Saunders; 2001.
22. Mee JF. Newborn dairy calf management. Vet Clin N Am Food Anim Pract 2008;24: 1–17.
23. Garry F, Adams R. Neonatal calf resuscitation for the practitioner. Agri-Pract 1996; 17:25–9.
24. Mee JF. Resuscitation of newborn calves: materials and methods. Cattle Pract 1994;2:197–210.
25. Brown LA. Improving the survival rate of dyspneic neonatal lambs. Vet Med 1987;82: 421–2.
26. Uystepruyst C, Coghe J, Dorts T, et al. Effect of three resuscitation procedures on respiratory and metabolic adaptation to extra uterine life in newborn calves. Vet J 2002;163:30–44.
27. Koterba AM. Identification of the high-risk neonate. In: Smith BP, editor. Large animal internal medicine. St Louis (MO): CV Mosby; 1990. p. 294.
28. Fecteau G, Smith BP, George LW. Septicemia and meningitis in the newborn calf. Vet Clin N Am Food Anim Pract 2009;25:195–204.
29. Lassen ED. Laboratory evaluation of plasma and serum proteins. In: Thrall MA, Campbell TW, DiNicola DB, editors. Veterinary hematology and clinical chemistry. Baltimore (MD): Lippincott Williams and Wilkins; 2007. p. 403–5.
30. Tyler JW, Parish SM, Besser TE, et al. Detection of low serum immunoglobulin concentrations in clinically ill calves. J Vet Intern Med 1999;13:40–3.
31. Tennant B, Baldwin BH, Braun RK, et al. Use of the glutaraldehyde coagulation test for detection of hypogammaglobulinemia in neonatal calves. J Am Vet Med Assoc 1979;174:848–53.
32. Rischen CG. Passive immunity in the newborn calf. Iowa State University Vet 1981; 12:60–5.
33. Stott GH, Marx DB, Menefee BE, et al. Colostral immunoglobulin transfer in calves. 2. Rate of absorption. J Dairy Sci 1979;62:1766–73.
34. Matte JJ, Girard CL, Seoane JR, et al. Absorption of colostral immunoglobulin-G in the newborn dairy calf. J Dairy Sci 1982;65:1765–70.
35. Bush LJ, Staley TE. Absorption of colostral immunoglobulins in newborn calves. J Dairy Sci 1980;63:672–80.
36. Devery JE, Davis CL, Larson BL. Endogenous production of immunoglobulin-IgG1 in newborn calves. J Dairy Sci 1979;62:1814–8.
37. Osburn BI, Maclachlan NJ, Terrell TG. Ontogeny of the immune system. J Am Vet Med Assoc 1982;181:1049–52.
38. Besser TE, Gay CC, Pritchett L. Comparison of three methods of feeding colostrum to dairy calves. J Am Vet Med Assoc 1991;198:419–22.
39. Miller M, Weber M, Neiffer D, et al. Use of commercially available plasma for transfusion in exotic ungulates. Conf. Proceedings American Association of Zoo Veterinarians. Milwaukee (WI): AAZV; 2002. p. 175.
40. Park Y, Wah GFW. Overview of milk of non-bovine mammals. Ames (IA): Blackwell; 2006.
41. Drackley JK. Calf nutrition from birth to breeding. Vet Clin N Am Food Anim Pract 2008;24:55–66.
42. Radostits OM. Veterinary medicine: a textbook of the diseases of cattle, sheep, pigs, goats, and horses. 10th edition. New York: Elsevier Saunders; 2007.
43. Heinrichs J. Rumen development in the dairy calf. Adv Dairy Technol 2005;17: 179–87.

Veterinary Pediatrics of Butterflies, Moths, and Other Invertebrates

Thomas C. Emmel, PhD[a,b,c,]*

KEYWORDS

• Butterflies • Moths • *Lepidoptera* • Eggs • Larva • Pupae

In the life cycle of invertebrate animals, the typical life history includes the egg and larval stage, which may be called the pediatric phases, representing development up to the point where the animal reaches adulthood with fully functional reproductive organs and full adult characteristics of morphology, coloration, physiology, and behavior. These typical immature or pediatric stages are found in both terrestrial and aquatic invertebrates.

In insects, by far the most speciose and numerically abundant invertebrates, the metamorphosis from egg to larva to adult may include a fourth stage, between the larva and the adult, called a pupa. This pupal stage, sometimes referred to as a "resting" stage because of its general immobility, is anything but resting. Instead, there is a dramatic breakdown and reorganization of larval tissues and cellular components into the new adult tissues and organs, all within a hard pupal shell. A complete metamorphosis (such as found in the butterflies and moths of the order Lepidoptera) will progress through egg, larval, pupal, and adult stages (**Figs. 1–6**). A species with an incomplete metamorphosis lacks the pupal stage and goes through the egg, larval (or nymphal), and adult progression.

Thus, from the viewpoint of a veterinarian, dealing with pediatric concerns, we are concerned with the maladies and problems associated with the egg, larval, and (if present) pupal stages of an insect or other invertebrate life history. Such veterinary medicine concerns are literally in their infancy. While much work has been done by economic entomologists focusing on ways to kill the development stages of crop pest insect species, there has been little effort until recently to consider ways to prevent diseases and other problems that beset early insect life cycle stages. However, with

The author has nothing to disclose.
[a] Department of Entomology and Nematology, University of Florida, Gainesville, FL 32611, USA
[b] McGuire Center for Lepidoptera and Biodiversity, Florida Museum of Natural History, PO Box 112710, Gainesville, FL 32611, USA
[c] Department of Zoology, University of Florida, Gainesville, FL 32611, USA
* McGuire Center for Lepidoptera and Biodiversity, Florida Museum of Natural History, PO Box 112710, Gainesville, FL 32611.
E-mail address: tcemmel@ufl.edu

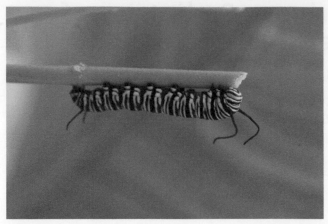

Fig. 1. The healthy, mature caterpillar of the Monarch butterfly (*Danaus plexippus*) will evidence a firm (taut) integument and extended front and rear tentacles, feeding every hour or so. A larva infected with pathologic virus or bacteria will have a flaccid skin and drooping tentacles, and may expel (via anus and mouth) a green liquid.

the rise since the 1980s of hundreds of commercial live butterfly display houses in England and subsequently across the world, there is now a demand for the application of care standards in zoos, aquariums, museums, and private enterprises such that butterflies and other invertebrate livestock have protection approaches similar to standards set already for birds, mammals, reptiles, amphibians, and fish (**Figs. 7** and **8**). The economic value of butterfly livestock alone raised each year on butterfly farms, and displayed to the public in specially constructed butterfly houses for the public to enjoy, now exceeds $1 billion. Thus, a longer adult life, greater chances of eggs and larvae and pupae surviving to the adult stage, and greater application of maintenance issues for the health of these adults for a proper diet and protection from disease will all contribute to healthy captive animals and thus more dynamic displays of these invertebrates. Additionally, a great increase in public interest in butterfly gardening at home, coupled with hand-rearing of local and exotic species at home for personal enjoyment and even companionship, makes it useful for a veterinarian to know the basic needs for maintaining healthy invertebrates through their life cycles, especially those of the butterflies and moths that people encounter and bring into their homes in their everyday activities or that are displayed in large numbers at public attractions.

This article reviews the factors that impact the health and survival of juvenile stages of butterflies and moths in particular, and what can be done to extend veterinarian care and advice to clients regarding invertebrate problems. As with vertebrates, in practice it is far easier to exercise prevention than to find and apply cures for these problems, at our present state of knowledge.

PROBLEMS WITH BUTTERFLY AND MOTH JUVENILE STAGES

In nature, the vast majority of eggs and larvae are destroyed by predators, parasitoides, and diseases that afflict them before they reach the adult stage. Of all the eggs a female can potentially produce, less than 1% will, on the average, survive to produce a replacement adult female and male. When a butterfly species is kept in

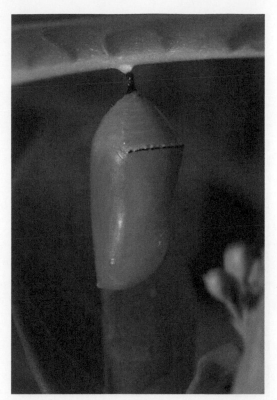

Fig. 2. During the first 8 days of the pupal stage of the Monarch butterfly, the ground color is a bright green, with gold spots and black trimming. The pupa is plump and firm to the touch. If any parasitic wasp or fly larvae are inside, the pupal shell will collapse during this period and turn black (but with no adult wings visible).

captivity as a pet or display animal, we have to eliminate these mortality factors that normally control the eventual adult numbers.[1] These problem areas can be summarized as follows.

Successful Mating of a Newly Emerged Female

Are the lighting, temperature, humidity, and enclosure volume of space adequate to meet the male and female needs to behave normally and respond to contact by a successful mating? With some 20,000 species of butterflies and perhaps 245,000 species of moths in the world, the breeder (and veterinarian) has to do considerable trial-and-error research to create the proper conditions, a search aided by review of the available literature and personal contacts with other breeders in the business or located in the home country of the species under investigation.

Provision of a Proper Host Plant for Egg Deposition

Is the client using a known host plant for that species, or can a related substitute plant species be provided? While this information may be gleaned from the available life history literature in some cases, it is lacking for most tropical species. It may be possible to suggest a locally available plant (eg, a lawn grass for grass-feeding

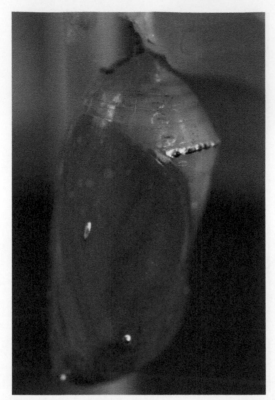

Fig. 3. In the penultimate day (normally day 9) of the pupal stage, a healthy Monarch pupa turns reddish brown, with black lines, where the miniature adult wings are developing on the sides of the front three-quarters of the pupa.

skipper or satyrid taxa, or privet [hedgerow] leaves for a silk moth species) as a substitute for more exotic or unavailable plants.

Care of the Mated Female so That She Will Live Long Enough to Deposit a Maximum Number of Eggs

Most butterfly and moth adults can be hand-fed once or twice daily with a 3:1 mixture of water and sugar (or honey). This procedure can be readily demonstrated to a client in an office setting. After mixing a 3:1 solution by shaking in a screw-cap vial, unscrew the cap, set it on a desktop, and fill the cap with the artificial nectar solution. Holding the 2 forewings together with thumb and forefinger, place the butterfly's front pair of legs in the edge of the cap's fluid. The proboscis (tongue) will immediately and automatically uncoil from under the head into the fluid, and the adult will start feeding. When she is finished (1–2 minutes), she will coil up her proboscis again and flex her wings or start to walk away. Pick her up with thumb and forefingers and return her to her cage over a potted host plant. If you do this daily, she will live as long as 1 month or longer, and lay hundreds of ova.

Protecting the Eggs

The egg stage may last as briefly as 5 days or as long as 9 months, depending on the species. During this period, the eggs can be kept on the plant covered by netting, or

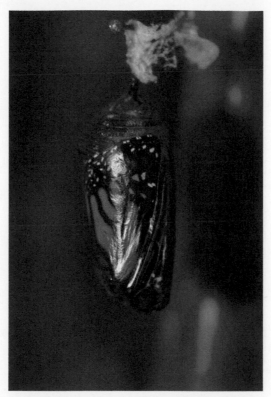

Fig. 4. On the last day (normally day 10) of the Monarch's pupal stay, the entire pupal shell becomes transparent (crystal-clear) and every structure of the developed adult can be seen, before the pupal sutures split apart and the adult emerges to expand and then harden its soft wings and body.

in a mesh or screen-covered jar, for protection from predators (eg, ants or stinkbugs) and parasitoids (eg, tiny wasps). It is possible to kill any microorganisms (bacteria and viruses) that might be on the outside of the egg shell, ready to infect the emerging larva, by dipping them briefly in a 2% bleach solution. But generally this step is not necessary unless your client has experienced a previous microorganism infection of larvae in the breeding colony, where spores may have been deposited on the outside of the female adult and transmitted via contact to the egg surface when laid.

Avoiding Food and Cleanliness Stresses for the Larvae

Be sure to always have sufficient larval host plant material on hand (and change food twice daily if putting leaves in a container such as a jar or plastic shoebox). If the larvae are feeding well all day (and even at night), they will grow faster and be healthier and be more resistant to infection. It is equally important to clean up all frass (larval droppings) and food remnants each time the food is changed. Using disposable paper towels or newspaper sheets in the bottom of a jar or plastic box helps to absorb excess humidity and larval droppings (throw this paper out twice a day). Clean desktop or counter surfaces by wiping with a 2% bleach solution.

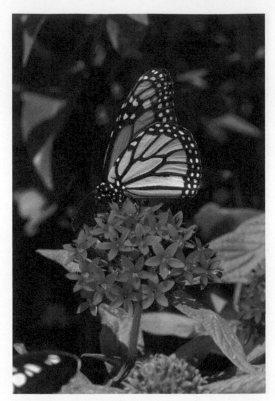

Fig. 5. The healthy adult Monarch butterfly on a Pentas flower, drinking nectar.

Protection of Larvae From Predators, Parasitoids, and Microorganisms

Protect the larvae from ants, stinkbugs, cockroaches, crickets, spiders, earwigs, ground beetles, slugs, mice, or other conceivable predators, at all times. The larvae should be kept on growing, potted host plants within finely meshed cages or plastic-sided containers at all times. If raised in jars or plastic boxes, the lids should fit tightly to keep out predators and parasites but a screened breathing opening is necessary to allow the passage of needed oxygen and waste carbon dioxide.

If larvae in one container become sick from bacteria or viruses, they will stop eating and then regurgitate their recent food as a greenish fluid, becoming flaccid. At that point, it is best to discard (burn or bury) that container's culture and soak the entire container in 50% bleach solution for 24 hours. While antibiotic solutions could be tried with the larvae that did not regurgitate yet in that culture container (larvae will drink droplets of dew or antibiotic-laced water from leaf surfaces), it is usually NOT worth the time and trouble to administer them unless the species is quite rare and the effort to save each caterpillar is paramount.

Quarantining new introductions to the culture room or building is the most effective way to prevent the entry of harmful organisms of all types. If this is followed by maintenance of a satisfactory food supply, environment for host plant growth, and prompt removal of any diseased organisms, the number of larvae surviving to the pupal and adult stages can reach 95% to 100% in your client's cultures.

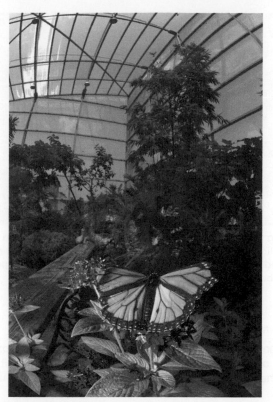

Fig. 6. The adult Monarch after 3 months of life in the Butterfly Rainforest at the Florida Museum of Natural History, showing a minor amount of normal wing wear from flying daily in and out of vegetation.

Pupal Care and Protection

If the larvae survive the vicissitudes of culture conditions and invading harmful organisms, they will stop feeding about 24 hours before pupation and go on a long walk to find a safe pupation site (generally a high location, under a protective leaf or stem, board, or stone). There the larva usually spins a silk pod on the substrate to attach its hind legs and perhaps (in swallowtails and sulfurs, whites, and their relatives) 2 silk threads from the thorax to the substrate. It molts its larval skin and reveals the pupa. This is a dangerous move for the larva, as it has to swing the cremaster hooks at the end of its abdomen around the wad of old larval skin and into this pad on the substrate, all within a fraction of a second. It is traumatic for the observer to see a fallen pupa that has been misshapen or injured by failure at this step, but there is no hope of recovery of the pupa if this sort of damage occurs. The new pupal skin will quickly harden, and if it is not perfectly formed, the developing butterfly days later will not emerge correctly and it will die.

The pupa may also die during metamorphosis to the new adult because of parasites or pathogens carried into the pupa from the previous larval stage. Prompt removal of the diseased (blackened) pupae is necessary so that other pupae are not affected.

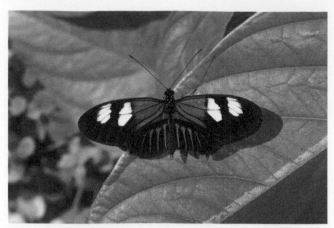

Fig. 7. A Longwing butterfly, *Heliconius erato*, commonly exhibited in butterfly display houses for the public. Adults live up to 5 to 6 months in such a protected environment, and the eggs, larvae, and pupae are rarely afflicted by disease. Hence, all the species of the genus *Heliconius* tend to be popular choices for display.

Emergence of the New Adult from the Pupae

At this stage of the complete metamorphosis process, the seams or sectional joints of the pupa split open along the thorax and head areas to permit the emergence (hatching) of the new adult from the pupal shell. The wings are small, highly folded (crumpled) pads.

The adult must quickly move outside the pupal shell and hang upside down to (1) pump hemolymph from the thorax into the hollow veins of the 4 wings and force their expansion and (2) allow the pull of gravity to aid in this wing expansion process. If the butterfly loses its grip with its legs and falls to the ground or floor of the container, it

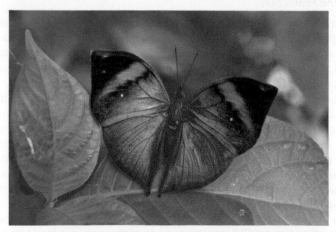

Fig. 8. The Asian leaf butterfly, *Kallima inachis*, is brilliant blue and orange on the upper surface but looks like a perfect dead leaf when the wings are folded and only the underside is exposed to view.

must be quickly put up again on a stick or leaf so it can hang, or its wings will harden in a crumpled state and it will die.

The butterfly expands its wings within 5 minutes and then must hang quiescently for 1 or 2 hours while the wing veins harden into struts and the hemolymph is withdrawn from the outer vein areas back to the thorax.

During this time, the butterfly will extend the 2 halves of its tongue (proboscis) and fit them together (side by side) into a hollow tube. This tube is then coiled under the head. If the butterfly fails to match up the 2 halves of its proboscis, they will harden separately and will not function as a drinking "straw" tube. Then the butterfly will die. Also at this stage, the antennae are extended into more-or-less straight protuberances, and the legs assume their final shape while the body hangs below them.

The butterfly may have a very fat abdomen for the first hour or so, and then expel (squirt out) a red fluid called meconium, representing all the waste products that accumulated inside the pupal shell as the larval tissues were broken down and re-built into the adult structures. This bloodlike fluid flow is normal and does not represent any injurious condition.

Adult Disease and Injuries

In the adult stage, few dangers are posed by microorganisms (aside from those that may accumulate on the outside of the body or wings and be transmitted to eggs laid by infected female adults). Some parasitic flies may likewise attack adult butterflies in tropical rainforests and lay their eggs on the adult's abdomen surface.

As far as veterinary advice goes on adult butterflies, most would pertain to injuries suffered such as broken wing veins leading to a flap of the wing hanging at an odd angle. One can repair such broken veins and broken wing edges using a tiny amount of contact cement and holding the immobilized wing in place for 30 seconds. This will restore normal wing lift and flight behavior, and the adult can live, feed, and even court and mate normally thereafter.

GENERAL COMMENTS ON TREATING PROBLEMS WITH BUTTERFLIES IN CULTURES AND DISPLAYS

Fresh food is essential for either larvae or adults. In the case of adults, nectar-feeding species need fresh flower nectar available daily or must be fed artificial nectar (3:1 mixture) once or twice daily, depending on amount of activity. Caterpillars should be raised on potted plants instead of cuttings whenever possible.

Cleanliness is essential for disease protection. Prevention by disinfection of the rearing environment can be done daily with an aerosol spray like Lysol (apply on cages or container surfaces for 30 seconds and remove with paper) or bleach (sodium hypochloride). Once infected, larvae must be removed and destroyed; they cannot be healed by any presently available methods. All larval frass and food debris must be removed at least daily or more frequently.

Keep larvae in uncrowded conditions. Excessive moisture from too many larvae or other high-humidity conditions will greatly increase the chances for larval disease.

Prevention of disease and parasites, along with removal of afflicted larvae from a client's culture are the only practical ways of caring for eggs, larvae, and pupae and the juvenile stages of adult butterflies at present. The consulting veterinarian must emphasize these points to concerned clients, whether private individuals or public displays and insect farms, in order to minimize the impacts of disease, parasites, and predators during the developmental stages or an invertebrate's life history.[2,3] For tarantulas, land crabs, or other noninsect invertebrates, the surface has hardly been scratched concerning veterinary care. But butterflies are being more carefully studied now by researchers as model organisms because of their economic importance to the institutions having large living displays and the sizeable worldwide investment in butterfly farms that provide living pupae and adults for live exhibits, wedding and funeral releases, and other novel uses. Considerable progress in both preventive care and healing techniques may be expected in the coming decades.

REFERENCES

1. Tampion J, Tampion M. The living tropical greenhouse: creating a haven for butterflies. Lewes, East Sussex (UK): Guild of Master Craftsman Publications; 1999. p. 76–7.

2. Boggs CL. Environmental variation, life histories, and allocation. In: Boggs CL, Watt WB, Ehrlich PR, editors. Butterflies: ecology and evolution taking flight. Chicago (IL): University of Chicago Press; 2003. p. 191–9.

3. Stamp NE. A temperate region view of the interaction of temperature, food quality, and predators on caterpillar foraging. In: Stamp NE, Casey TM, editors. Caterpillars: ecological and evolutionary constraints on foraging. London: Chapman & Hall; 1993. p. 478–98.

Basics of Macaque Pediatrics

Andrea Saucedo, MV, RLATG*, Pablo R. Morales, DVM, DACLAM

KEYWORDS

• Macaque pediatrics • Infants • Nonhuman primate

Pediatrics involves a philosophy of comprehensive and continuing health care dedicated to the survival and subsequent development of a strong, healthy, and well-adjusted infant. Macaque pediatrics plays an essential role in any setting whether it be a research setting, display, or conservation purposes. This article focuses on macaque infants born and raised in captivity. Different approaches may be taken into consideration when working with other species of nonhuman primates. There are multiple parameters that are measured and evaluated from birth in order to detect problems early and maximize health. Nonhuman primates are usually born during the night or early hours of the morning. In an ideal situation, from this moment onward, they are cared for by their mothers until weaning.

PHYSICAL EXAMINATION

The evaluation of health status in any infant macaque is based on the collection of information obtained through observation and ancillary diagnostic techniques, followed by the systematic recording of these facts. Many parameters are measured in the newborn macaque, including the placental examination, which involves weighing, measuring, and counting the number of placental discs. The insertion, number of vessels, and length of the umbilical cord are also evaluated. If the cord is too long, there is an increased risk for strangulation; if it is too short, there could be difficulty passing through the canal. Part of the initial examination of the infant macaques is the ocular evaluation, which can reveal bilateral papillary membranes along with unilateral or bilateral remnants, which can last up to 2 weeks.

A more thorough examination involves the Simian Apgar scoring system, which is used in rhesus and cynomolgus macaques, and scores are obtained at 1, 5, and 10 minutes after birth. The respiratory rate, heart rate, muscle tone, skin color, alertness, responsiveness, and rectal temperature are rated. The rating is from 0 to 2 points for all categories, for a maximum of 12 points[1] (**Table 1**). Blood collection is generally done to allow evaluation at birth and at 2, 4, and 8 months of age on a routine basis. Additional evaluation is done as needed.

The authors have nothing to disclose.
Department of Veterinary Medicine, The Mannheimer Foundation Inc, 20255 SW 360 Street, Homestead, FL 33034, USA
* Corresponding author.
E mail address: asaucedo@mannheimerfoundation.org

Vet Clin Exot Anim 15 (2012) 289–298
http://dx.doi.org/10.1016/j.cvex.2012.03.006
1094-9194/12/$ – see front matter © 2012 Published by Elsevier Inc.

Table 1
Apgar scoring system

	0 Points	1 Point	2 Points	Points Totaled
Activity (muscle tone)	Absent	Arms and legs fixed	Active movement	
Pulse	Absent	<100 bpm	>100 bpm	
Grimace (reflex irritability)	Flaccid	Some flexion of extremities	Active, motion (sneeze, cough, pull away)	
Appearance (skin color)	Blue, pale	Body pink, extremities blue	Completely pink	
Respiration	Absent	Slow, irregular	Vigorous cry	

Severely depressed 0-3
Moderately depressed 4-6
Excellent condition 7-10

Anthropometrics

Head measurements (biparietal and occipitofrontal diameters, head circumference), hand and foot lengths, chest and arm circumferences, skin-fold thickness, crown-rump length, and total body weight are taken periodically to document normal growth rate.[2] A smaller measurement could be due to a short gestation, a mother small in size, prenatal psychosocial stress, or an abnormal growth rate. Infants born at less than 150 gestational days are defined as premature. Larger measurements are seen in cases of gestational diabetes or have also been related to larger females.

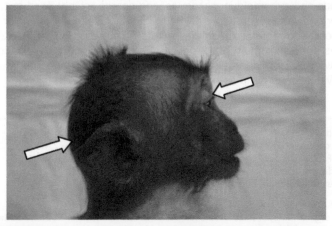

Fig. 1. Head length.

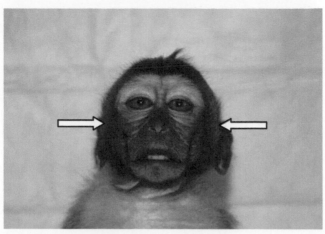

Fig. 2. Head width (Frankfurt plane).

Head length
With spreading calipers, measure the length from the area between the eyes to the occiput (**Fig. 1**). If the animal is disturbed by the procedure, it can be blindfolded. Read the measurement while the calipers are in place.

Head width or biparietal diameter
With the spreading calipers, measure between the 2 widest points of the skull; the landmarks are just above and in front of the ears (**Fig. 2**). Feel for these points first and then replace your fingers with the calipers.

Foot length
Place the monkey's heel flush with the base of the sliding scale (**Fig. 3**). Center the foot directly over the scale, with toes aligned and completely extended. Read the length from the end of the longest toe, excluding the nail. For accuracy in reading, you must be positioned directly over the scale.

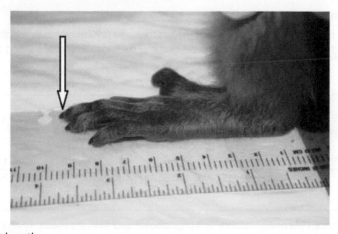

Fig. 3. Foot length.

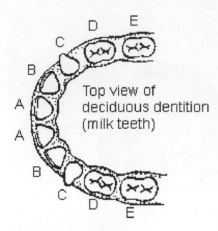

A—central incisors or I1
B—lateral incisors or I2
C—canines
D—first molar
E—second molar

Eruption of teeth generally develops in such order.

Fig. 4. Macaque dentition.

Dentition

The dentition of a macaque is a typical primate dentition. It is diphyodont and heterodont (**Fig. 4**).
The dental formula for the deciduous dentition is:
I 2/2 C 1/1 M 2/2
The permanent dentition has a dental formula:
I 2/2 C 1/1 PM 2/2 M 3/3.

Physical Growth and Body Weights

Females are relatively light (465 g) in comparison to males (490 g), yet their weight averages out at around 2 months of age until the end of the growth period (**Tables 2** and **3**).

Table 2													
Body weight (in grams) of female macaques in relation to chronologic age taken month by month, up to 1 year of age													
Age in Months	Birth	1	2	3	4	5	6	7	8	9	10	11	12
Mean body weight (grams)	465	600	770	915	1085	1255	1415	1560	1680	1815	1940	2070	2185

Data from Watts E. Collected anatomical and physiological data from the rhesus monkey. In: Bourne GH, editor. The rhesus monkey, vol I: anatomy and physiology. New York: Academic Press; 1976. p. 13–4.

Table 3
Body weight (in grams) of male macaques in relation to chronologic age taken month by month, up to 1 year of age

Age in Months	Birth	1	2	3	4	5	6	7	8	9	10	11	12
Mean body weight (g)	490	620	790	960	1125	1295	1450	1590	1725	1840	1950	2070	2195

Data from Watts E. Collected anatomical and physiological data from the rhesus monkey. In: Bourne GH, editor. The rhesus monkey, vol I: anatomy and physiology. New York: Academic Press; 1976. p. 13–4.

Neurobehavioral Examination

Include evaluation of the following reflexes:

- Blinking: closes eyes in response to bright light
- Babinkski: toes extend upward when foot is struck
- Crawling: the infant begins crawling motion when placed on its abdomen
- Moro's reflex: the infant throws the arms out, head back, and opens hands with a rapid change of position
- Palmar and plantar grasps: digits curl around a finger
- Startle: closing of hands after sudden loud noise.

NEONATAL BEHAVIORS

Very little control is normally required from a macaque newborn, except for maintaining contact with its mother and orienting its head and mouth to the mother's nipple at approximately 1 to 2 hours from birth. In addition to such basic clasping, grasping, and suckling reflexes, neonate macaques exhibit a number of other responses, including various postures, gross locomotion and limb movements, manipulation of objects, and visual/auditory orienting reactions.[3]

PRENATAL PSYCHOSOCIAL STRESS

Prenatal psychosocial stress can lead to decreased birth weights, impaired neuromotor development, decreased levels of exploratory behavior, as well as abnormal social behavior. Situations capable of producing the latter include loud noises, disruption of social groups as a result of relocation, and dominance relations during pregnancy.[4]

REARING EXPERIENCES

Infant macaques have been reared under the following circumstances.[4]

- Total isolation: This is not the ideal circumstance since it can produce abnormal behavior and inappropriate social behavior.
- Surrogate only: These infants have access to an inanimate terry cloth covered mother, yet still do not present normal social behavior.
- Partial isolation: These infants, although housed singly, are able to view, hear, and smell the surrounding monkeys.
- Peer only: These infants are separated from their mother at birth and placed in a nursery with others of a comparable age. This atmosphere seems to develop a social behavior in which they play, groom, and show aggression toward their peers. They still tend to cling onto others.
- Surrogate peer: These infants receive continuous exposure to inanimate mothers and are exposed to infants of their same age for no more than 2 hours per day. This decreased the rate of infants clinging onto one another.

- Mother only: Infants reared this way develop a full range of species-specific behaviors.

NURSERY REARING: HANDREARING

The ideal circumstance for an infant macaque is the care and nurturing it receives from its mother and the attention it receives from its family and additional group members. Unfortunately, situations do occur that necessitate the removal of an infant from its parents.

Common Causes of Hand Rearing

- Prolonged illness of infant/failure to thrive
- Prolonged illness of mother
- Maternal neglect/abandonment experience
- Abuse of offspring/aggression toward infant may be propagated by family members or unrelated members of the troop
- Experimental design.

NUTRITIONAL NEEDS

Macaques require vitamin C in their diets as well as folic acid, selenium, chromium, and fluoride. A specially formulated milk for primates (Primilac; Bio-Serv, Frenchtown, NJ, USA) provides all the nutrients and has more calories than its human counterparts. Other types of infant formulas used include Isomil Similac Soy, Similac with iron (Abbott, Columbus, OH, USA), and Enfamil Prosobee (Mead Johnson and Company, Evansville, IN, USA).

FEEDING SCHEDULES

During the first 24 hours of life, while the suction/swallow reflex is assessed and strengthened, the newborn is fed 5% to 10% dextrose water. After this first day, it can then begin with a milk replacer. Mix half of the amount of milk replacer and the other half dextrose water until gradually reducing the percentage of dextrose water in the first 2 to 5 days of life. By day 5, infants can be fed every 2 to 3 hours during the first month of life. Afterward, the infants can begin using self-feeders. At 2 to 4 weeks after birth, solid foods can be introduced if milk alone is not satisfying its appetite. Timing varies from individual to individual. Primate commercial diet (biscuits) can be softened in a fruit juice or offered with a quarter slice of fruit (ie, orange). This is done to prevent the deterioration of vitamin C with plain water. By 12 weeks of age, biscuits should no longer be softened (**Table 4**).

Table 4							
Recommended fruits and vegetable portions by age							
Age/Species	**Orange**	**Apple**	**Banana**	**Cucumber**	**Green Pepper**	**Celery**	**Carrots**
Young infants (2–4 mo)	<1/8 slice	<1/8 slice	½-inch sliver	Not for young infants	Not for young infants	Not for young infants	Not for young infants
Older infants (>4 mo)	1/8 slice	1/8 slice	1-in sliver	1-inch sliver	1/8 slice	½-inch piece	½-inch piece

GAVAGE FEEDING

Infants born at around 150 gestational days are considered to be at increased risk for aspiration pneumonia. A 3.5 to 5 French infant feeding tube, orogastric tube, or nasogastric tube can be used for gavage feeding. The amount to feed is 10 to 20 mL/kg of body weight. Prior to passing of the tube, it should be measured externally to calculate the distance from the oral cavity to the stomach. Measure to immediately past the last rib. Then mark the tube in order to prevent excessive introduction of the tube causing irritation or damage to the stomach mucosa. As in any species, the tube must be passed in a careful manner in order to avoid the trachea. To facilitate this, the patient is placed in a sitting posture with the neck extended. Gavage feeding is best achieved with 2 handlers unless the infant is unresponsive or conscious and not too feisty, in which case it may be a 1-person task.

HUSBANDRY CONSIDERATIONS

Isolettes should be cleaned on a daily basis. The product used to clean in our facility is dilute Roccal-D Plus (Pfizer, New York, NY, USA). After cleaning, the isolette is rinsed thoroughly with tap water. Fleece blankets should be provided for enrichment as they provide not only warmth but also comfort to the infant. Washable toys and clean bedding should be maintained at all times. When the transition from incubator to cage occurs, a dry system is ideal. The dry system consists of cleaning cages without using water on a daily basis. Bedding is placed on the pan to absorb bodily fluids (urine, feces, etc). It is used to prevent wetting debilitated animals and avoid aerozolization. Different types of bedding exist including but not limited to alfalfa pellets, corn cob, and paper. One inconvenience with this system is its labor intensiveness due to the fact that cages need to be changed on a weekly basis, and cage bars are to be scrubbed with a brush.

The temperature setting for the isolette/incubators during the first 2 weeks of life should be 93° to 95°F. Then it is decreased to 90° to 93°F during the second and fourth weeks of life. It is important to maintain an adequate humidity (30%–70%).[5] Increased humidity can exacerbate problems associated with temperature extremes.

DEVELOPMENT/SOCIAL NEEDS

Psychological well-being in primates depends on appropriate infant development. There are multiple methods of defining this term. Reproductive success (reproductive behavior, fertility, prenatal adequacy, parturition, and parental care) is generally considered the strongest indicator of psychological well-being in captive nonhuman primates.[6] Last, the optimum situation in which a primate should develop is one that permits the infant to remain with its biological mother through weaning in the company of a species-normal social group.

WEANING

Macaque mothers wean their infants at the age of about 1 year. Natural weaning is a gradual process by which the mother, over a period of several weeks or months, discourages her infant to suck on her breasts. Once the mother stops nursing the infant, the young usually remains in the maternal group at least until prepuberty. Under confinement conditions, artificial weaning is an abrupt event that takes place several months prior the normal biological age of weaning. Artificial weaning or permanent mother–infant separation prior to natural weaning is a common husbandry practice in monkey breeding colonies in United States.

Primatologists repeatedly have emphasized the deleterious effects of early maternal separation on juvenile macaques. The International Primatological Society recommends that "the young monkey should not normally be separated from its mother at an early age (ie, at 3–6 months) but should remain in contact for one year to 18 months, in most species. There is unlikely to be any greater productivity through early weaning, in seasonally breeding species, such as rhesus monkeys. Even in non-seasonal breeders (such as long-tailed macaques), any slight increase in productivity must be offset against the resulting behavioural abnormalities of the offspring."[7]

PREVENTATIVE MEDICINE
Immunizations and Deworming

This protocol usually begins at 3 months of age with deworming. Multiple anthelminthics are used. These include ivermectin (Ivomec, Merial, Duluth, GA, USA) given at 0.2 mg/kg (200 μg/kg) subcutaneously and fenbendazole (Panacur; Bio-Serv, Frenchtown, NJ, USA) tablets given at 50 mg/kg. The immunizations start at 6 months, as well as the tuberculin testing. The standard dose of mammalian tuberculin (Colorado Serum Company, Denver, CO, USA) is 0.1 mL intradermal injection on the upper eyelid margin, which is essential for the health surveillance of any macaque colony (**Table 5**).

Table 5				
Immunizations and deworming				
Product/Procedure	**Age**	**Injection Site**	**Route**	**Frequency**
Ivermectin	3 mo	Scruff	Subcutaneously	Every 6 mo
TB testing	6–12 mo	Upper eyelid	Intradermally	Every 6 mo
Rabies	6–12 mo	Right flank	Subcutaneously	Every 3 y
Tetanus	6–12 mo	Right leg	Deep intramuscularly	Every 5 y
Serology	9 mo	Femoral vein	Intravenously	6 mo–1 y

Rabies vaccine (Rabvac 3, Fort Dodge, IA, USA) and tetanus toxoid (Fort Dodge) are also given.

Most Common Health Problems

Problems will most often occur in infant macaques. These include hypothermia, hypoglycemia, dehydration, and, in less prevalence, trauma. Trauma to the infants is usually not caused purposely but is circumstantial. This simply occurs as the infant is clinging onto its mother and is caught in between fighting individuals. Another common condition associated with clinging is digit trauma caused by the constant wrapping of hair around the fingers.

The most common scenario of a health problem is finding a baby down in its enclosure or very weak and unable to grasp onto its mother. Upon arrival to triage, a thorough physical examination is performed, ensuring that the infant is weighed, skin turgor on the chest is checked to determine the hydration, and the rectal body temperature is read, followed by an examination of the eyes, ears, nose, and mucous membranes. The majority of times the body temperature is too low to register when you introduce the thermometer (digital with flexible tip [Jorvet, Jorgensen Labs, Loveland, CO, USA] rectally, with a probe cover [Sunmark, McKesson, San Francisco, CA, USA; Vet-Temp, Advanced Monitors Corporation, San Diego, CA, USA]). This is the most accurate method from a medical point of view, because it comes closest to the core body temperature. On occasions, an ear thermometer has been used but its efficacy has not been determined. A blood glucose reading should be done in order to rule out hypoglycemia. The sample can be collected from one of the digits or ischial callosity. In cases of hypoglycemia, the infant can be offered or fed via orogastric tube a warm 5% to 10% dextrose solution.

In infants less than 6 months of age, the most frequent cause of death is attributed to respiratory system issues, which include respiratory distress syndrome, pulmonary atelectasis, and pneumonia. The next most common cause of death in animals less than 1 year old is gastrointestinal disease. This problem may be due to many causes and is extremely difficult to totally erradicate. Iatrogenic diarrheas are often caused by destruction of normal enteric flora. Some of the most common causes of diarrhea are of bacterial origin, including *Shigella* spp, *Campylobacter* spp, *Yersinia* spp, *Salmonella* spp, and *Escherichia coli*. Viral and parasitic infections are encountered less frequently. Among the viral pathogens, rotavirus has been reported. Parasitic causes of diarrhea include cryptosporidiosis, *Enterobius, Trichuris,* and *Strongyloides*. Mycotic conditions are also reported with *Candida albicans* (thrush) as the most common agent.

Stress can also be a precursor to infectious diarrheas and other diseases. Another common diarrhea in infants results from dietary changes or overconsumption of milk or feed. It can sometimes be corrected by limiting available food or diluting formula as required. Lactose intolerance is common in neonates and can be reversed by substituting with soy-based formulas.

SUMMARY

It is clear that raising infants with their mothers and family group is ideal for their appropriate development. When this is not feasible, it is necessary to try to detect abnormalities beforehand and avoid circumstances that can be detrimental to the animal's social and reproductive behavior. It is of great importance to try to simulate as much as possible an environment adequate enough to develop a species-specific behavior. Multiple measurements and parameters exist to evaluate macaque infants. Although infants are vulnerable to multiple health problems, with effort and dedication and 24-hour care, many times these can be corrected.

REFERENCES

1. Hendrickx AG, Dukelow WR. Breeding. In: Bennett T, Abee C, Henrickson R, editors. Nonhuman primates in biomedical research: biology and management. Atlanta (GA): Elsevier; 1995. p. 360–1.
2. Ferrier C. Standard operating procedure for anthropometrics of infant nonhuman primates. 2002. Available at: depts.washington.edu/iprl/sop/anthropometricSOP.pdf. Accessed March 21, 2012.
3. Watts E. Collected anatomical and physiological data from the rhesus monkey. In: Bourne GH, editor. The rhesus monkey, vol I: anatomy and physiology. New York: Academic Press; 1976. p. 13–4.
4. Novak MA, Sackett GP. The effect of rearing experiences: the early years. In: Sackett GP, Ruppentahal GC, Elias K, editors. Nursery rearing of nonhuman primates in the 21st century. New York: Springer Science + Business Media; 2006. p. 5–16.

5. National Research Council. Guide for the care and use of laboratory animals. 8th edition. Washington, DC: National Academies Press; 2011.
6. Novak MA, Suomi SJ. Social interaction in nonhuman primates: an underlying theme for primate research. Lab Anim Sci 1991;41:308–14.
7. Reinhart V. Artificial weaning of Old World monkeys: benefits and costs. J Appl Anim Welfare Sci 2002;5(2):151–6.

Overview of Veterinary Chiropractic and Its Use in Pediatric Exotic Patients

Marilyn M. Maler, DVM[a,b,c,*]

KEYWORDS

• Veterinary • Chiropractic • Exotic animals • Pediatric

VETERINARY CHIROPRACTIC HISTORY, EDUCATION, AND CERTIFICATION

Techniques and theories of veterinary chiropractic have been adapted from human chiropractic, which has been documented back to many ancient civilizations, including Greek, Chinese, Indian, Japanese, Roman, and Egyptian. The first modern human chiropractic school was opened in 1897 by Daniel David Palmer and later became known as Palmer School of Chiropractic.[1] At the Palmer School of Chiropractic, D.D. Palmer treated animals with chiropractic care partly to disprove critics' claims that positive effects of chiropractic care seen in humans were a placebo effect. Veterinary chiropractic was formalized in the late 1980s when Dr Sharon Willoughby, holding doctorates in both veterinary medicine and chiropractic medicine, initiated a postgraduate educational program, which later became known as Options for Animals College of Animal Chiropractic.[2]

Veterinary chiropractic, like human chiropractic, is a skill that must be taught in a comprehensive and logical manner, using both didactic and practical hands-on training. It is strongly recommended that any veterinarian or chiropractor interested in adjusting animals attend one of the veterinary chiropractic schools approved by the American Veterinary Chiropractic Association (AVCA) and the International Veterinary Chiropractic Association (IVCA). The approved postgraduate animal chiropractic education programs are listed in **Box 1**. Only licensed doctors of veterinary medicine or doctors of chiropractic are admitted into these postgraduate programs. After successful completion of an approved animal chiropractic course, the doctor can apply for certification through the AVCA or IVCA. These courses teach basic adjusting techniques of dogs and horses. Once the practitioner is proficient in those species,

The author has nothing to disclose.
[a] Options for Animals College of Animal Chiropractic, Wellsville, KS 66092, USA
[b] Chi Institute of Chinese Medicine, Reddick, FL 32686, USA
[c] SunSpirit Farm and Veterinary Services, Inc., 18815 NW County Road 239, Alachua, FL 32615, USA
* SunSpirit Farm and Veterinary Services, Inc., 18815 NW County Road 239, Alachua, FL 32615.
E-mail address: canter@windstream.net

Vet Clin Exot Anim 15 (2012) 299–310
doi:10.1016/j.cvex.2012.03.001
1094-9194/12/$ – see front matter © 2012 Elsevier Inc. All rights reserved.

Box 1
Approved Postgraduate Animal Chiropractic Education Programs

Options for Animals College of Chiropractic, Kansas, USA

Healing Oasis Wellness Center, Wisconsin, USA

Parker College of Chiropractic, Texas, USA

Veterinary Chiropractic Learning Center, Ontario, Canada

---

where spinal anatomy and facet joint angles have been studied and published, he or she can safely extrapolate and apply that knowledge base and skill to other species. While there are no animal chiropractic courses that teach exotic animal adjusting techniques, there are many private practice veterinarians, chiropractors, and zoo practitioners who have adapted basic veterinary chiropractic techniques and developed skills to adjust exotic species.

VERTEBRAL SUBLUXATIONS: ROLE IN THE THEORY AND PRACTICE OF CHIROPRACTIC

Vertebral subluxation is at the core of chiropractic theory, and its detection and correction are central to chiropractic practice. The chiropractic term "vertebral subluxation" has caused much misunderstanding between the chiropractic profession and the medical and veterinary professions. The medical and veterinary definition of "subluxation" describes an orthopedic view of partial or incomplete joint dislocation. Obviously, chiropractors do not treat these true pathologic subluxations. A chiropractic vertebral subluxation is a decreased or abnormal range of motion (ROM) of a facet joint where there is no disruption of articular surfaces.[3] While there are many forms of body work and joint mobilization techniques, chiropractors are the only health care practitioners trained to diagnose and correct a chiropractic vertebral subluxation. Vertebral subluxations are diagnosed by manually testing the ROM of every facet joint of the patient. Once diagnosed, the subluxation is corrected by a chiropractic manipulation or adjustment, which is a high-velocity, low-amplitude dynamic thrust using a specific contact point and line of correction with the intention of freeing the restricted joint and improving the ROM of the joint.[4]

The early chiropractic definition of "vertebral subluxation" was a very limited view that focused mainly on a simplistic and static structural theory. Historically, "bone out of place" and "pinched nerve" were common phrases used to describe a subluxation complex and, although incorrect, they are still often heard. The true effects of a vertebral subluxation are not limited to a local or even segmental decreased ROM. The term "vertebral subluxation complex" (VSC) has evolved to help describe the widespread dysfunction secondary to a subluxation. The definition of "subluxation" accepted by all human chiropractic colleges is "A complex of functional and/or structural and/or pathological articular changes that compromise neural integrity and may influence organ system function and general health."[3] The contemporary model of VSC is a dynamic and complex model that includes abnormal joint motion, associated soft tissue changes, and vascular, inflammatory, and biochemical changes. The neurologic manifestations associated with a VSC are often the most observable and problematic to the patient and may be felt or observed far distant from the offending subluxation.[5,6]

Vertebral Subluxation Effects on Spinal Mobility and Regional Range of Motion

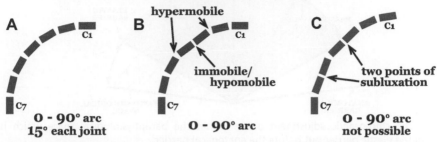

Fig. 1. A representation of cervical vertebrae C1 through C7 and associated motion units. For simplicity it is assumed that each motion unit contributes equally to the regional ROM. (*A*) When all motion units of a region have a normal ROM, each motion unit contributes to the overall ROM of that region. (*B*) When a subluxation or restriction is present in a motion unit, the motion units above and below the restricted area must contribute a larger than normal individual ROM in order for the regional ROM to remain unaffected. (*C*) When multiple subluxations are present, adjacent motion units may not be able to increase their individual ROM enough and the regional ROM will be decreased.

Effects of Vertebral Subluxations on Spinal Motion Units

A motion unit consists of vertebral bodies of adjacent vertebrae and all the associated soft tissues, including ligaments, muscles, blood vessels, nerves, and joints. It is the facet joints and disk that allow for movement of a motion unit in the spine, but it is the muscles that initiate and direct the motion. The connective tissues surrounding a respective motion unit are then affected by the motion, or lack of motion. A VSC of one or more facet joints will cause decreased or abnormal range of motion of that motion unit. This altered motion then causes dysfunction of the associated soft tissues and spinal nerve as they pass through the intervertebral foramen (IVF). In addition to affecting the associated spinal nerve, the VSC also has detrimental effects on the motion units adjacent to it. Because the spine acts as an integrated unit, a restriction of motion in one area leads to increased motion in adjacent areas. When a motion unit is hypomobile or nonmobile, the motion units adjoining it will become hypermobile in order to compensate. **Fig. 1**A demonstrates how all the joints evenly share the amount of motion of a spinal region when there are no subluxations creating fixation or restriction. Conversely, in **Fig. 1**B, motion units adjacent to subluxations are subject to an abnormal increased ROM to allow the entire spinal region normal, complete ROM despite the subluxated motion units that are not able to contribute their portion of the total ROM. The body recognizes this hypermobility of adjacent motion units as abnormal and attempts to stabilize the hypermobile area, causing restriction and eventually immobilization of that motion unit and setting up a cycle of continuing pathology. Eventually, if enough motion units become subluxated, restricted, or immobilized, the adjacent vertebrae can no longer compensate enough and overall mobility of that spinal region is decreased as is demonstrated in **Fig. 1**C.[5–8]

RANGE OF MOTION AND THE CHIROPRACTIC ADJUSTMENT

Every joint, including facet joints have an ROM that can be divided into 3 zones: physiologic, paraphysiologic, and pathologic (**Fig. 2**). The physiologic ROM of a

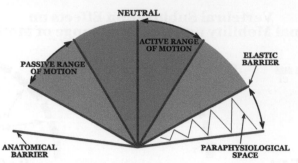

Fig. 2. The chiropractic adjustment occurs within the paraphysiological space which is beyond the elastic barrier but before the anatomical barrier.

motion unit consists of the active ROM and the passive ROM. The active ROM is the amount of motion, in a specific direction, that the bones of a motion unit should be able to move actively, initiated by voluntary muscle activity. The passive ROM is located at the end of active ROM and is the additional amount of motion that the motion unit can move passively, as a result of an outside force. Joint mobilization, as is used in other forms of manual physical therapy, occurs within the physiologic ROM. The limit of a motion units' physiologic ROM, active plus passive ROM, is determined by the semirestrictive elastic barrier consisting of periarticular ligaments and other connective tissue that binds the unit. Beyond the elastic barrier, but before the anatomic barrier, is the paraphysiologic ROM or zone. The paraphysiologic zone is the area in which chiropractic joint manipulation and treatment occurs. The anatomic barrier defines the absolute end ROM; any motion beyond the anatomic barrier is considered to be in the pathologic zone and would result in injury and damage to the joint or motion unit. Correct chiropractic treatment never crosses the anatomic barrier.[5,6,9]

The differences between mobilization and manipulation are more important than the ROM in which they are employed. The physiologic effects of manipulation versus mobilization are significant. In humans, chiropractic manipulation has been shown to immediately relieve local spontaneous myoelectric activity, while mobilization does not.[9] This unique special effect of manipulation makes chiropractic adjustments especially helpful in spinal and paraspinal pain relief.

Joint cavitation produces the characteristic popping or cracking sound elicited during a manipulation or adjustment when the elastic barrier of resistance is overcome. This sound is caused by vapor and gas bubbles formed within joint fluid by a sudden local reduction of pressure. An audible crack or pop is not a requirement for a successful adjustment, however.[9,10]

REVIEW OF SPINAL ANATOMY SPECIFIC TO CHIROPRACTIC MEDICINE

The spine is divided into anatomic regions: cervical, thoracic, lumbar, and sacrum with pelvis. The number, shape, size, and orientation of vertebrae in each section vary by species, but all vertebrae provide protection for the spinal cord as its travels through the vertebral foramen. Spinal nerves with their associated afferent sensory and efferent motor branches split off the spinal cord and pass through the IVF. The location of the IVF in relation to the facet joint (also called zygapophyseal or apophyseal joints) can be seen in **Fig. 3**. Altered, decreased, or absent motion of a facet joint constitutes a vertebral subluxation. The facet joint in a motion unit is formed

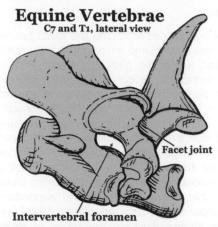

Equine Vertebrae
C7 and T1, lateral view

Facet joint

Intervertebral foramen

Fig. 3. The facet joint consists of the caudal articular facet of the cranial vertebrae and the cranial articular facet of the caudal vertebrae. The facet joint angle is key to successful chiropractic diagnosis and treatment. Note the proximity of the IVF and the facet joint.

by the cranial articular process of the caudal vertebrae and the caudal articular process of the cranial vertebrae. Facet joints are gliding synovial joints oriented at oblique angles to the spine. The angle of facet joints varies by species and spinal region.[11,12] The facet joint angle orientation is important to the veterinary chiropractor because adjustments must be performed in the plane of the normal joint angle, called the angle or line of correction.[10]

CONTEMPORARY HYPOTHESIS OF VERTEBRAL SUBLUXATION COMPLEX AND ASSOCIATED NEURAL DYSFUNCTION

There have been various hypotheses to explain the neural dysfunction associated vertebral subluxations including but not limited to: nerve compression hypotheses, aberrant spinal reflex hypotheses, joint dysafferentation, visceral disease simulation, and decreased axoplasmic transport.[13] It is beyond the scope of this report to discuss the details of most hypotheses, but due to its long history and prominence in chiropractic theory, nerve compression hypothesis is important to understand and is summarized as follows.

The spinal nerve is in an anatomically precarious position as it passes through the IVF. Because of the bony boundaries of the IVF, any constriction in or around the IVF predisposes to compression/impingement of the exiting spinal nerve, dorsal root ganglion, and vessels. Additionally, spinal nerve roots are more easily compromised than peripheral nerves due to their less abundant protective epineurium and poor lymphatic drainage. Spinal nerve roots are extremely sensitive to pressure, and as little as 10 mm Hg produces a significant conduction block and alteration of nerve function. As little as 5 to 10 mm Hg pressure will block venous blood flow within the IVF to the spinal nerve roots, resulting in venous stasis and swelling that are considered to be a significant cause of nerve root compression. The nerve compression hypothesis maintains that spinal nerve roots become compressed secondary to spinal biomechanical derangements and spinal nerve root compression can cause clinically significant biomechanical and physiologic changes.[13]

CHIROPRACTIC RESEARCH

While there are several hypotheses regarding the exact pathways that subluxations effect physiologic changes, human and animal clinical studies that demonstrated the presence of widespread neurologic and physiologic effects after experimentally induced subluxations compared to control or sham groups. Descriptive clinical research studies have demonstrated improvement in gastrointestinal, respiratory, urogenital, reproductive, musculoskeletal, and cardiovascular disorders after chiropractic treatment.[14] Inhibition of myoelectric activity of the upper gastrointestinal tract of rabbits was induced after a chiropractic lesion was simulated.[15] With other factors equal, duodenal ulcers in humans healed faster when chiropractic care and manual soft tissue therapy were added to standard treatment.[16] A clinical trial showed a statistically significant decrease in systolic and diastolic blood pressures of hypertensive patients after chiropractic treatment and supported the hypothesis that hypertensive patients show a short-term reduction in blood pressure after chiropractic treatment.[17] These studies illustrate the types of research that have been conducted and refute the common argument that there is no research supporting effectiveness of chiropractic care. Chiropractic research is in its infancy compared to traditional medicine largely due to lack funding and proprietary interest in chiropractic as well as historical staunch opposition from the American Medical Association and other medical groups. Despite these setbacks, chiropractic medicine received international attention when a 1994 report by the US Agency for Healthcare Policy and Research ranked spinal manipulation/adjustment in the first two treatment options (among 22 treatment options) for acute low back pain.[18]

SPECIAL CONSIDERATIONS FOR EXOTIC PEDIATRIC PATIENTS

Exotic animal veterinarians are well versed in adapting standard veterinary practices to meet the specific needs of their uncommon patients; chiropractic care for exotics is no different. Veterinary chiropractic schools teach basic adjusting techniques on dogs and horses; the practitioner will need to modify those techniques based on their patients' needs. Because of the vast skeletal differences of exotic animals, it is beyond the current scope to describe species-specific adjusting techniques. The study of dissected spines and particularly the facet joints of species of interest will aid the practitioner but is not necessary. The vertebral formulas for many mammalian, avian, and reptilian pet species are summarized by Dr R.D. Ness.[19] He finds that mammals have the most consistent vertebral formulas, and reptiles, the least documented. In fact, all mammals, with the exception of 2-toed sloths and manatees, have 7 cervical vertebrae.[20]

The key to becoming a proficient, skillful veterinary chiropractor of any species is to motion palpate as many "normal" animals as possible. One cannot recognize altered, decreased, or absent motion of a VSC without the comparison of normal motion. It is the facet joints that determine the direction of motion of the motion units and thus the line or angle of correction that the veterinary chiropractor will use. Ness reports that motion palpating and adjusting cats is good practice for chiropractic care of ferrets as both have similar-feeling, highly mobile spines (Robert Ness, DVM, personal communication, 2011). The author finds that her equine chiropractic experience allows her to competently adjust exotic hoofstock such as llamas and deer. Dr De Grasse, DC, finds that palpating and motioning the joints above and below the subluxation helpful in determining the correct line of correction when dealing with an unfamiliar species (Jacqueline De Grasse, RN, DC, personal communication, 2011). She also uses radiology, performed by the referring veterinarian, when appropriate to help locate areas of spinal misalignment. Feeling for heat resulting from inflammation is also helpful to locate subluxations.

De Grasse and Ness explain that the major difference in treating pediatrics of any species versus a mature animal is the presence of an exaggerated ROM afforded their joints due to immature ligamentous structures supporting the joint (Jacqueline De Grasse, RN, DC, personal communication, 2011; Robert Ness, DVM, personal communication, 2011). Both doctors also stress that pediatric patients require much less force to adjust compared to mature animals. Human pediatric resources also advise that the normal relative hypermobility of pediatric patients be appreciated by the chiropractor.[7,21] Ness believes that chiropractic care improves the survival and development of many runts and "swimmers" of various species (Robert Ness, DVM, personal communication, 2011). A swimmer is a neonate that cannot stand or walk at the appropriate development stage and lies with limbs splayed out similar in appearance to a turtle. Etiology of swimmer syndrome is unknown, but conservative treatment with passive and active manual therapy techniques such as assisted standing/walking, massage of limbs, and stimulation of feet to initiate a withdrawal reflex is often successful. Since other manual therapies appear to help, adding chiropractic care to the treatment plan for neonates with swimmer syndrome is logical.

Safety and Contraindications

When performed by a properly trained and skilled doctor, chiropractic care is a very safe modality, but it should always be preceded by a thorough physical examination and indicated diagnostic tests. Chiropractic care is contraindicated in animals with neoplasia, fractures, and acute disc disease. There is some concern that chiropractic adjustments may speed the metastasis of neoplasia when performed on patients with cancer. Once fractures are stabilized or acute disc disease has subsided, afflicted patients can receive chiropractic care.[22]

Use of Anesthesia or Tranquilization

The use of anesthesia or sedation is rare in the chiropractic treatment of domestic animals, but may be necessary for many exotic species. The animal must be relaxed enough to allow the doctor to motion and manipulate its spine. Adjustments cannot be forced upon a patient; muscle tension will not allow a proper adjustment if the animal is resistant. Its use does require the doctor to be aware that the motion will not feel the same as in a fully conscious patient. Normal protective mechanisms and reflexes are diminished or absent and extra care must be taken not to adjust beyond the anatomic barriers of the joint of or in an incorrect line of correction.

SPECIES-SPECIFIC CONSIDERATIONS IN CHIROPRACTIC CARE OF EXOTIC PETS AND BIRDS
Small Mammals

Rabbits are probably the exotic animal species most frequently presented for chiropractic care and fortunately are also relatively easy to motion palpate and adjust. Some rabbits can be adjusted while on an examination table, but many feel more secure when held close to the doctors body (**Fig. 4**). They also tend to have positive clinical responses from therapy. The combination of very powerful hindlimb muscles and a delicate spine make rabbits prone to spinal trauma and chiropractic subluxations, with the L6-7 motion unit the most common site for injury. Hindlimb paresis and paralysis are common presenting complaints in rabbit medicine and are often improved or completely reversed when chiropractic care is added to traditional

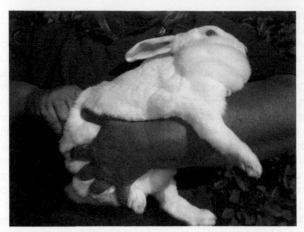

Fig. 4. Many doctors prefer to adjust small exotic animals while securing them against their own body rather than on an examination table.

medical therapy. Radiographic examination is necessary prior to chiropractic care if trauma is known or suspected.

Chiropractic treatment can increase spinal mobility in rabbits with spondylosis. Because hopping is a rabbit's mode of locomotion, there is an exaggerated flexion and extension of the lumbar vertebrae and lumbosacral region. Consequently, there tends to be calcification of the ventral longitudinal ligament and occasionally the dorsal longitudinal ligament of these areas as the body attempts to stabilize the hypermobile areas. Chiropractic care can relieve some of the fixations secondary to mineralization of these ligaments but will not reverse the calcification.

Rabbits are often presented for chiropractic care suffering from torticollis secondary to otitis media, parasitic migrans, or cerebrovascular accidents. The torticollis often remains even after the primary underlying condition is appropriately treated. No matter the underlying cause, rabbits with torticollis often respond positively to chiropractic treatment, benefiting from a reduction in severity of head tilt and decreased neurologic deficits. Cervical subluxations are a common finding in these rabbits, but hyoid and temporomandibular joint fixations need to be considered also.[19,23]

Ferrets are also good candidates for chiropractic treatment for several reasons. Ferrets are very similar to cats with regard to spinal mobility, so a doctor experienced in adjusting cats may easily transfer that skill to ferret chiropractic. Although squirmy, ferrets can be distracted by offering Laxatone (Vétoquinol USA Inc., Fort Worth, TX, USA) during the chiropractic examination. Stabilizing the ventral abdomen of the ferret by draping it over the underside of the practitioners forearm, with the ferret's forelimb and thorax in the practitioner's palm, and adjusting with the free hand is the preferred method of restraint.[19,24]

Adrenal gland disease is a common finding in older ferrets and leads to generalized muscle atrophy, including the epaxial and hypaxial muscles responsible for spinal support. This leaves the afflicted ferret predisposed to vertebral subluxations, especially of the lumbar spine. Ferrets are predisposed to several forms of neoplasia that would contraindicate chiropractic care, including spinal lymphoma, osteosarcoma, and chodroma.[19,24]

There are several internal medicine diseases of ferrets and rabbits that may be cured or ameliorated by chiropractic care. Following the logic of research previously cited that showed decreased myoelectric activity of the upper gastrointestinal tract of rabbits when a chiropractic subluxation was simulated, some cases of gastrointestinal stasis of rabbits may be the result of a chiropractic subluxation disrupting the nerve supply to the gastrointestinal tract and thus may be corrected through chiropractic treatment.[15] Similarly, a chiropractic subluxation causing dysfunction of nerves supplying the bladder may cause urinary incontinence or bladder atony, depending on the spinal area that is compromised and if sympathetic or parasympathetic fibers are involved. Ferrets suffering with symptoms of inflammatory bowel disease may be helped also.[19,23,25]

Guinea pigs have a few peculiar characteristics that make them good candidates for chiropractic care. The pubic symphysis of the female will fuse, resulting in a narrowed pelvic canal, at approximately 7 to 8 months if not bred. If bred after fusion of the pubic symphysis, or if obese, the guinea pig is at an increased risk of dystocia. Any neonate delivered after dystocia should be evaluated for chiropractic lesions.[19]

Guinea pigs may suffer from scurvy if adequate exogenous vitamin C is not supplied. Symptoms include spondylosis and arthritis, especially of the lumbar spine and costochondral junctions and joint inflammation. Along with standard protocol of vitamin C supplementation and anti-inflammatory drugs, chiropractic treatment is indicated after the joint inflammation has subsided.[19]

Reptiles

Due to the absence of a diaphragm and the subsequent lack of defined thorax and abdomen, the spinal regions of reptiles are termed presacral, sacral, and caudal instead of cervical, thoracic, lumbar, and caudal as in mammals. The chiropractic lesions encountered in reptiles originate primarily from poor husbandry, inadequate nutrition, or trauma. Lizard or tortoise species that have recovered from metabolic bone disease and have residual scoliosis can be managed with chiropractic care. Metabolic bone disease, also known as nutritional secondary hyperparathyroidism, causes very fragile bones that are easily fractured. Spondylosis and spinal deviation are common secondary effects of metabolic bone disease that are amenable to spinal adjustments. Radiographs are necessary to rule out fractures and assess the health of the skeletal system before proceeding with chiropractic therapy.[19] Ness and De Grasse report success treating egg-bound snakes (Jacqueline De Grasse, RN, DC, personal communication, 2011; Robert Ness, DVM, personal communication, 2011).

Avian

To allow for flight, birds have evolved several distinct skeletal characteristics to be considered. Whether or not flighted, all are bipedal and have forelimbs that are modified into wings. Compared to other animals, the avian skeleton is very lightweight, constituting only 4.4% of the body mass of a pigeon.[19] On radiographs, avian long bones have normally thin cortices, a feature that would indicate osteoporosis in a similar size mammal. This is due in part to the invasion of avian air sac system into the medullary cavity of various pneumatic bones including the humerus, coracoid, sternum, pelvis, and vertebrae, and the femur and scapula in some avian species.[25]

Also, a large portion of the avian vertebral column is fused. The synsacrum is formed by the fusion of lower thoracic, lumbar, sacral, and caudal vertebrae. The terminal caudal vertebrae fuse to form the pygostyle, and cranial thoracic vertebrae fuse to form the notarium. These areas of fusion leave only 3 areas that are mobile and subject to chiropractic subluxations: the highly mobile cervical region, vertebrae between the notarium and synsacrum, and vertebrae between the synsacrum and pygostyle.[19]

Chiropractic care is indicated for several avian conditions. Trauma incurred by flying into windows or mirrors is a common cause of cervical vertebral subluxation. Dystocia and egg binding due to deficient smooth muscle function may be relieved by chiropractic care if there is impingement/compression of the spinal nerves supplying the necessary smooth muscles.[19] Feather picking is considered a behavioral problem triggered by stress or environmental factors.[26]

Chiropractic theory may explain some cases of feather picking differently. Paresthesia is the sensation of tingling, burning, pricking, or numbness of one's skin that can arise from irritation of spinal or peripheral nerves supplying the affected area. Formication is a form of paresthesia that describes the sensation that of insects crawling on or under the skin. Paresthesia of hands and fingers is a common symptom of humans suffering from cervical vertebral subluxations and is often relieved by regular chiropractic care. Some veterinary chiropractors believe that the excessive grooming behaviors associated with canine lick granulomas and avian feather picking are sometimes the animals' reactions to paresthesia or formication of the afflicted area and report improvement, if not complete resolution, of symptoms with chiropractic treatment.

Hoofstock

Depending on size, exotic hoofstock can be adjusted with chiropractic techniques used for canines or equines. If tame, many larger exotic hoofstock species can be adjusted similarly to horses; with little or no restraint. Stocks are often used to adjust cattle and may be used for large exotic hoofstock also. De Grasse finds that when adjusting species with long, highly flexible necks, such as llamas, traction applied to the cervical vertebrae assists chiropractic treatment (Jacqueline De Grasse, RN, DC, personal communication, 2011). Birth trauma can cause vertebral subluxations in any mammalian species. In hoofstock, this may cause upper cervical subluxation that results in difficulty or inability to properly position their neck to nurse. Gastrointestinal issues, especially colic-type symptoms of newborns, may respond favorably to chiropractic treatment added to standard medical therapy. After chiropractic care, human newborns are often relieved of persistent colic symptoms that have not responded to standard medical therapy. Upper cervical subluxations, possibly sustained during the birth process, are the most common finding in human newborns with colic.[27]

REVIEW OF CHIROPRACTIC CARE OF PEDIATRIC EXOTIC PATIENTS

Chiropractic care is occasionally sought for treatment of residual effects from traumatic accidents such as a pockets pets that are dropped or birds that fly into windows, but chiropractic treatment has much more to offer veterinary practice. While the positive effects of chiropractic on musculoskeletal conditions are the most obvious, one should not forget chiropractic care in the treatment plan for visceral or behavioral conditions. Rabbits, ferrets, and birds are commonly treated by veterinary chiropractors, but any animal with a spine may present with disorders secondary to vertebral subluxations. When performed by a trained and skilled doctor, chiropractic care is very safe and can correct vertebral subluxations that can cause neurologic dysfunction and have widespread detrimental effects on our patients' health.

REFERENCES

1. Willis J. Forerunners of the chiropractic adjustment. In: Cleveland CS, Redwood D, editors. Fundamentals of chiropractic. St Louis: Mosby; 2003. p. 3–13.

2. Bockhold H, Eschbach D. The history of animal chiropractic. In: Options for Animals College of Animal Chiropractic Basic Course Notes, vol 1. Wellsville (KS): Options for Animals; 2005. p. 2–5.
3. Cleveland CS. Vertebral subluxation. In: Cleveland CS, Redwood D, editors. Fundamentals of chiropractic. St Louis (MO): Mosby; 2003. p. 129–37.
4. Bockhold H, Eschbach D. What is animal chiropractic? In: Options for Animals College of Animal Chiropractic Basic Course Notes, vol 1. Wellsville (KS): Options for Animals; 2008. p. 1–4.
5. Eschbach D. General biomechanics. In: Options for Animals College of Animal Chiropractic Basic Course Notes, vol 1. Wellsville (KS): Options for Animals; 2008. p. 1–6.
6. Leach RA. Segmental dysfunction hypothesis. In: Butler J, Napora L, Schwartz AK, editors. The chiropractic theories: principles and clinical applications. Philadelphia: Lippincott Williams & Wilkins; 1994. p. 43–52.
7. Anrig CA. Spinal examination specific specific spinal and pelvic adjustments. In: Anrig CA, Plaugher G, editors. Pediatric chiropractic. Baltimore (MD): Williams & Wilkins; 1998. p. 323–423.
8. Kirkaldy-Willis WH. Managing low back pain. New York: Churchill and Livingstone; 1983. p. 82.
9. Leach RA. Integrated physiological model for the VSC. In: Butler J, Napora L, Schwartz AK, editors. The chiropractic theories: principles and clinical applications. Philadelphia: Lippincott Williams & Wilkins; 1994. p. 373–86.
10. Scaringe JG, Cooperstein R. Chiropractic manual procedures. In: Cleveland CS, Redwood D, editors. Fundamentals of chiropractic. St Louis (MO): Mosby; 2003. p. 257–89.
11. Coughlin P. Spinal anatomy. In: Cleveland CS, Redwood D, editors. Fundamentals of chiropractic. St Louis: Mosby; 2003. p. 45–88.
12. Coughlin P. Spinal neurology. In: Cleveland CS, Redwood D, editors. Fundamentals of chiropractic. St Louis (MO): Mosby; 2003. p. 91–116.
13. Cleveland CS. Neurologic relations and chiropractic applications. In: Cleveland CS, Redwood D, editors. Fundamentals of chiropractic. St Louis (MO): Mosby; 2003. p. 155–81.
14. Masrasky CS, Todres-Masarskey M. Somatovisceral research. In: Cleveland CS, Redwood D, editors. Fundamentals of chiropractic. St Louis (MO): Mosby; 2003. p. 531–54.
15. Deboer K, Schutz M, McKnight ME, et al. Acute effects of spinal manipulation on gastrointestinal myoelectric activity in conscious rabbits. Manual Med 1988;3:85–94.
16. Pikalov AA, Kharin VV. Use of spinal manipulative therapy in the treatment of duodenal ulcer. J Manipul Physiol Ther 1992;17:310.
17. Yates RG, Lamping DL, Abram NL, et al. Effects of chiropractic treatment on blood pressure and anxiety: a randomized, controlled trial. J Manipul Physiol Ther 1988;11: 484.
18. Bigos S, Bowyer O, Braen G, et al. Clinical Practice Guideline No. 14: acute lower back pain in adults. AHCPR Publication No. 95-0642. Rockville (MD): Agency for Health Care Policy and Research, Public Health Services, US Dept of Health and Human Services; 1994.
19. Ness RD. Anatomic and physiologic considerations in chiropractic care of birds and exotic pets. In: Proceedings of the 2010 American Veterinary Chiropractic Association. Bluejacket (OK): American Veterinary Chiropractic Association; 2010.
20. Bockhold H, Eschbach D. General anatomy. In: Options for Animals College of Animal Chiropractic Basic Course Notes, vol 1. Wellsville (KS): Options for Animals; 2005. p. 5–10.

21. Alcantara J, Anrig CA, Plaugher G. Pediatrics. In: Cleveland CS, Redwood D, editors. Fundamentals of chiropractic. St Louis (MO): Mosby; 2003. p. 349–61.
22. Lauretti WJ. Comparative safety of chiropractic. In: Cleveland CS, Redwood D, editors. Fundamentals of chiropractic. St Louis (MO): Mosby; 2003. p. 561–78.
23. Ness RD. Chiropractic care of rabbits. In: Proceedings of the 2010 American Veterinary Chiropractic Association; 2010.
24. Ness RD. Chiropractic care for exotic pets. Exotic DVM 2000;2.1:15–8.
25. Smith BJ, Smith SA. Radiology. In: Altman RB, Club SL, Dorrestein GM, et al, editors. Avian medicine and surgery. Philadelphia: WB Saunders; 1997. p. 170–98.
26. Davis C. Behavioral problems. In: Altman RB, Club SL, Dorrestein GM, et al, editors. Avian medicine and surgery. Philadelphia; WB Saunders; 1997. p. 653–7.
27. Tanaka ST, Martin CJ, Thilbodeau P. Clinical neurology. In: Anrig CA, Plaugher G, editors. Pediatric chiropractic. Baltimore (MD): Williams & Wilkins; 1998. p. 479–611.

Introduction to Traditional Chinese Veterinary Medicine in Pediatric Exotic Animal Practice

Huisheng Xie, DVM, MS, PhD[a],*, Christine Eckermann-Ross, DVM, CVA, CVCH[b]

KEYWORDS

- Traditional Chinese veterinary medicine • Exotics
- Pediatrics • Herbals
- Acupuncture • Aquapuncture

The term "exotic animals" refers to any animals that are not domesticated. Exotic pets are nondomesticated animals or strikingly unusual pets. They continue to increase in popularity and a larger variety of species are frequently presented to veterinarians for treatment. Exotic animals include (1) small mammals including rabbits, ferrets, hamsters, guinea pigs, and rats; (2) birds; (3) zoo animals including elephants, tigers, bears, giant pandas, monkeys, and giraffes; (4) reptiles and amphibians; (5) marine mammals, ornamental fish, sea lions, and seals; and (6) others such as ruminants including llamas, alpacas, bovines, sheep and goats, and any other wildlife.

Traditional Chinese veterinary medicine (TCVM) has been used to treat domestic livestock and horses in China for nearly 3000 years.[1,2] In TCVM, disease is considered as disharmony in interaction among the internal organs and between the interior of the body and exterior of the environment. The TCVM fundamental principles are to identify imbalance of *Yin-Yang* of the body and to use herbs, acupuncture, *Tui-na*, food therapy, or a combination to restore the balance.[3] *Yin* refers to the parasympathetic system such as resting, storage of energy, decreased heart rate, vasodilation, etc. *Yang* is like the sympathetic system physiologic activities, discharge of energy, increased heart rate, vasoconstriction, etc. In general, *Yin* refers to cooling and nourishing energy, while *Yang* is warming and functioning energy. *Tui-na* is the Chinese medical manipulation and is especially useful for pediatrics.

TCVM has now been used in many exotic animals, including birds,[4] rabbits,[5] elephants,[6] monkeys,[7] giant pandas,[8] tigers,[9] jaguars,[10] tortoise,[11] and many others.[12]

Disclosure: Dr Huisheng Xie is one of the owners of Jing-tang Herbal, Inc.
[a] Small Animal Clinical Sciences, University of Florida College of Veterinary Medicine, PO Box 100126, 2015 SW 16th Avenue, Gainesville, FL 32608-0136, USA
[b] Avian & Exotic Animal Care, PA, 8711 Fidelity Boulevard, Raleigh, NC 27617, USA
* Corresponding author.
E-mail address: xieh@ufl.edu

Table 1		
TCVM basal energetics in zoo animals		
TCVM Energetic	Species	Comments
Yang	Birds	Yang compared to all other animals
	Tigers and wild cats	Yang compared to the majority of other mammals
	Bears	Yang compared to most mammals
	Pigs	Yang compared to most omnivorous mammals
	Monkeys	Yang compared to most mammals
Mixed Yin and Yang	Giant pandas	Yin compared with bears, but Yang compared to other herbivores
	Elephants	Yang compared to camelids
	Camelids	Yin compared to other mammals but Yang compared to sheep/goats
	Sheep/goats	Yin compared to most mammals but Yang compared to cows
	Rats and mice	Yin compared to most mammals, but Yang compared to rabbits
	Marine mammals, sea lions, and seals	Yin compared to most mammals, but Yang compared to reptiles and amphibians
	Ornamental fish	Yin compared to most mammals, but Yang compared to reptiles and amphibians
Yin	Reptiles	Yin compared to most animals
	Amphibians	Yin compared to most animals
	Rabbits	Yin compared to most mammals
	Cows	Yin compared to other mammals

Data from Xie H, Trevisanello L. Application of traditional Chinese veterinary medicine in exotic animals. Reddick (FL): Jing Tang Publishing; 2011.

Some species (reptiles) can be treated with acupuncture, while others (giant pandas and dolphins) may be treated with herbs alone. However, most species can be treated with a combination of acupuncture, herbs, *Tui-na,* and food therapy. This article focuses on general principles and case examples of how to use TCVM in these exotic animals.

TCVM ENERGETIC THEORY AND APPLICATION

It is important to know species energetics and TCVM patterns to treat as noninvasively as possible. Exotic animals commonly have different basal energetic qualities than our domestic companion animals (**Table 1**). In general, mammals can be either *Yin* or *Yang.* Avian species are more *Yang,* while reptiles and amphibians are more *Yin.*

Yang *Species*

The core of TCVM is the balance of *Yin* and *Yang.* In general, a *Yin* method (gentle and quiet) is required to approach *Yang* species. The *Yang* species are prone to having heat or *Yin* deficiency (often with a red, dry tongue). Cool or cold foods and herbs may be used to balance the *Yang* constitution.

Yin *Species*

The *Yin* species are prone to having cold/damp patterns, and *Qi/Yang* dDeficiency (often with a pale, wet tongue). They enjoy quiet environments; thus, a *Yin* method (gentle and quiet) is also required to approach *Yin* species. Warm foods and herbs may be used to balance the *Yin* constitution.

ACUPUNCTURE
Where Are Acupuncture Points Located?

Historically, veterinary acupuncture initially started in horses, and then was also used in other species including cattle, camels, pigs, dogs, cats, rabbits, and birds. Professor Chuan Yu (1924–2005), the most important figure in modern TCVM history, devoted his life to teach TCVM and study veterinary history and acupuncture. After 50 years teaching TCVM and research experience and the consultation of more than 500 books and literature including ancient veterinary acupuncture texts, Professor Yu, along with the contribution of his colleagues, wrote *Zhong Gao Shou Yi Zhen Jiu Xu* (*Chinese Veterinary Acupuncture and Moxibustion*), which was published in 1995. The book has described in detail 173 acupoints in horses, 103 acupoints in cattle, 85 acupoints in domesticated pigs, 77 acupoints in camels, 76 acupoints in dogs, 74 acupoints sheep and goats, 51 acupoints in rabbits, 32 acupoints in cats, 34 acupoints in chickens, and 35 acupoints in ducks.[13] It serves as a base and root for most of modern veterinary acupuncture books in both Chinese and other foreign languages. The majority of acupoints can be transpositioned from the Yu's model to these exotic animals based on anatomy. Some acupoints, such as those in rats and mice, have been better identified from recent research using these species.[14,15]

What Acupuncture Points Should Be Used?

It is simple. Use the acupoints that your patient lets you use! In general, needle or acupressure *Bai-hui* or GV-20 first if available, and then start with acupoints around the neck, shoulders, and back. If *Bai-hui* or GV-20 is not available (your patient is too tall or does not allow you to use), other acupoints to calm the *Shen* (mind) are *An-shen*, GV-17, BL-10, GB-21, PC-6, and HT-7 (**Table 2**).

Three Tips for Successful Acupuncture Treatment

1. Distal acupoints on the paws and toes are "no-touch" zones in many species.
2. Begin with simple point combinations (3–6 acupoints) and *do not use too many needles.*
3. Keep the first acupuncture treatment short, like 5 to 10 minutes.

Which Acupuncture Techniques to Use?

Dry-needle and aquapuncture are most commonly used. Electroacupuncture can be used for nerve damage. Acupressure and laser can also be used.

HERBAL TREATMENT
Dosage

Dosage depends on different herbal formulas, severity of disease(s), size of animal, and individual variation. Thus, it is very difficult to give general guidelines for all exotic animals. **Table 3** is intended to provide a baseline for dosing exotic animals.

Table 2
Most commonly used acupoints in exotic animals

Clinical Conditions	Acupoints	Comments
Anorexia	*Shan-gen, Jian-wei*, BL-20/21	Used in lizards, cows, goats, sheep, pigs, rabbits, horses, dogs, cats
Diarrhea	GV-1, SP-6, BL-20/21	Used in lizards, cows, goats, sheep, pigs, rabbits, horses, dogs, cats
Vomiting/nausea	PC-6, GB-34, CV-12	Used in goats, sheep, rabbits, dogs, cats
Constipation	GV-1, BL-25, ST-37	Used in turtles, whales, goats, sheep, rabbits, horses, dogs, cats
Seizure	*Da-feng-men, Nao-shu*, LIV-3	Used in rabbits, horses, dogs, cats
Behavioral problems	*An-shen, Da-feng-men*, HT-7, GV-20	Used in birds, rabbits, horses, dogs, cats
High fever	GV-14, *Er-jian*	Used in elephants, goats, sheep, rabbits, horses, dogs, cats
Nasal discharge/congestion	LI-20, *Bi-tong, Long-hui*	Used in birds, goats, sheep, rabbits, horses, dogs, cats
Asthma/dyspnea	*Ding-chuan*, CV-22, CV-17	Used in goats, sheep, rabbits, pigs, horses, dogs, cats
Cough	*Ding-chuan*, CV-22, LU-7	Used in pigs, birds, goats, sheep, rabbits
Coma	GV-26, PC-6/TH-5, KID-1, PC-8, HT-9	Used in pigs, goats, sheep, rabbits, horses, dogs, cats
Bleeding	*Tian-ping*, GV-5/6/7	Used in goats, sheep, rabbits, horses, dogs, cats
General weakness	LI-10, ST-36	Used in lizards, goats, sheep, rabbits, tigers, bears, birds, horses, dogs, cats
Immune boosting	LI-4/11, GV-14, ST-36	Used in lizards, goats, sheep, rabbits, tigers, bears, birds, horses, dogs, cats
Spider/snake bite	GV-14, *Er-jian, Wei-jian*, LI-10, ST-36, TH-5, LI-4, LIV-3, GB-34/41	Used in dogs, sheep

Data from Xie H, Trevisanello L. Application of traditional Chinese veterinary medicine in exotic animals. Reddick (FL): Jing Tang Publishing; 2011.

Forms and Administration

- *Capsule:* This is the easiest way to medicate carnivores as capsules can be hidden in meat chunks.
- *Powder:* Top dressing of loose herbal powder can be used for elephants, giraffe, bovines, equines, and birds. Herbal powder mixed with water can be given as an enema in llamas, alpacas, goats, and sheep. Powder hidden inside the feeder fish can easily be given to dolphins and other marine mammals. Powdered

Table 3
Herbal dosage in exotic animals

Species	Oral Dosage Per Animal	Oral Dose Per Body Weight
Elephant/camel/giraffe	100–300 g bid	0.1–1 g/10 kg bid
Equine family (zebra, mule, donkey)	10–60 g bid	0.1–1 g/10 kg bid
Bovine	10–60 g bid	0.1–1 g/10 kg bid
Llamas, alpacas	5–15 g bid	0.1–1 g/10 kg bid
Goats/sheep	5–10 g bid	0.2–1 g/10 kg bid
Pigs	5–10 g bid	0.2–1 g/10 kg bid
Tiger, lion, jaguar	2–10 g bid	0.2–1 g/10 kg bid
Giant panda	5–15 g bid	0.2–1 g/10 kg bid
Dolphins	7–15 g bid	0.3–0.6 g/10 kg bid
Rabbits	0.5–1 g bid	0.3–0.6 g/1 kg bid
Rats/hamsters/ferrets/guinea pigs	0.05–0.2 g bid	0.5–1 g/1 kg bid
Chicken and duck	0.05–0.2 g bid or 1%–2% concentration in mediated diet	0.5–1 g/1 kg bid
Small birds (<2 kg) including African Grey parrots and cockatoos	0.05–0.2 g bid	0.5–1 g/1 kg bid
Most lizards, most turtles, amphibians		0.2–0.5 g/1 kg SID or bid
Some larger reptiles, most snakes		0.2–0.5 g/1 kg EOD or SID
Fish	1% concentration in medicated diet	

Abbreviations: EOD, every other day; SID, once daily.

formulas can also be mixed with compounding agents or hand feeding formulas for oral administration in most species. A medicated gel diet can be prepared and fed to fish.

- *Teapill:* Teapills can be used for birds.

Which Herbal Formula Should Be Selected?

In any medical system, effective treatment of disease hinges on accurate, complete diagnoses. This places *Bian Zheng*, the TCVM diagnostic system, as the most important part of medical practice. *Bian*, which is differentiation and identification, and *Zheng*, which is a type or pattern of illness, together indicate that the TCVM diagnostic system relies on pattern differentiation. **Table 4** lists Chinese herbal formulas for most commonly seen conditions and patterns in exotic animals.

TCVM IN PEDIATRICS

In general, one of the most common problems occurred in infants and pediatrics is gastrointestinal disorder. These young animals require more energy intake proportionally. For example, puppies require more energy proportionally than adult canines until they reach 80% of their adult body weight. However, overfeeding overwhelms the gastrointestinal system, leading to spleen *Qi* deficiency. Spleen *Qi*

Table 4
Most common herbal formulas in exotic animals

Clinical Condition	TCVM Pattern	Herbal Formula	Comments
General pain management	Qi-blood stagnation	Body Sore[a] or *Shen Tong Zhu Yu*	Has been used in elephants, giraffes, tigers, goats, sheep, llamas, alpacas, pigs, rabbits, birds, and dolphins in addition to horses, dogs, and cats
General weakness	Qi deficiency	Four Gentlemen[a] or *Si Jun Zi Tang*	Has been used in elephants, giraffes, tigers, goats, sheep, pigs, rabbits, reptiles, and birds in addition to horses, dogs, and cats
Immune deficiency	Lung/spleen Qi deficiency	*Wei Qi* Booster[a]	Has been used in elephants, bears, tigers, goats, sheep, pigs, rabbits, birds, reptiles, ornamental fish, and dolphins in addition to horses, dogs, and cats
Rear weakness	Qi deficiency with stagnation	*Bu Yang Huan Wu*	Has been used in elephants, giraffes, tigers, goats, sheep, pigs, rabbits, and birds in addition to horses, dogs, and cats
	Qi + Yin deficiency	Hindquarter Weakness[a]	Has been used in elephants, giraffes, tigers, bears, goats, sheep, pigs, rabbits, and birds in addition to horses, dogs, and cats
Paresis or paralysis	Qi-blood stagnation at spine	Double P #2[a]	Has been used in tigers, bears, horses, dogs, and cats
Cervical stiffness or wobblers	Cervical Qi-blood stagnation	Cervical Formula[a]	Used in giraffes, tigers, and birds in addition to horses, dogs, and cats
Gastric ulcers	Stomach Yin deficiency	Stomach Happy[a]	Has been used in dolphins, ferrets, birds, llamas, horses, dogs, and cats
Stomatitis or severe gastric ulcer	Stomach heat	Jade Lady[a] or *Yu Nu Jian*	Has been used in dolphins, llamas, horses, dogs, and cats
Chronic watery diarrhea	Spleen Qi deficiency	*Shen Ling Bai Zhu*	Has been used in giant pandas, birds, rabbits, goats, ferrets, small rodents, and sheep in addition to horses, dogs, and cats

(continued on next page)

Table 4
(continued)

Clinical Condition	TCVM Pattern	Herbal Formula	Comments
Poor appetite or anorexia	Spleen *Qi* deficiency with stomach *Qi* stagnation	Qi Performance[a]	Has been used in elephants, goats, sheep, llamas, alpacas, pigs, rabbits, small rodents, sugar gliders, reptiles, and birds in addition to horses, dogs, and cats
Vomiting or nausea	Stomach *Qi* rebeling	Happy Earth[a]	Has been used in dolphins, rabbits, horses, ferrets, small rodents, birds, reptiles, dogs and cats
Chronic dry cough	Lung *Yin* deficiency	Lily Combination[a] or *Bai He Gu Jin*	Has been used in goats, sheep, llamas, alpacas, pigs, rabbits, ferrets in addition to horses, dogs, and cats
Urinary incontinence	Kidney *Qi* deficiency	*Jin Suo Gu Jing*	Has been used in, bovines, horses, dogs, and cats
Seizure	Internal wind	*Di Tan Tang*	Has been used in birds, monkeys, rabbits, ferrets, rats, dogs, cats, and horses
Behavior issues	*Shen* disturbance	*Shen* Calmer[a]	Has been used in rabbits and, birds in addition to horses, dogs, and cats
Renal failure	Kidney *Qi/Yang* deficiency	*You Gui Wan*	Has been used in elephants, goats, sheep, llamas, alpacas, pigs, rabbits, and birds in addition to horses, dogs, and cats
	Kidney *Yin* deficiency	Rehmannia 6[a] or *Liu Wei Di Huang*	Has been used in elephants, goats, sheep, llamas, alpacas, pigs, rabbits, ferrets, reptiles, amphibians, and birds in addition to horses, dogs, and cats
	Kidney *Qi* + *Yin* deficiency	Rehmannia 11[a]	Has been used in elephants, goats, sheep, llamas, alpacas, pigs, rabbits, and tigers in addition to horses, dogs, and cats
Heart failure	Heart *Qi* deficiency	Heart *Qi* Tonic[a]	Has been used in goats, sheep, llamas, alpacas, pigs, rabbits, and birds in addition to horses, dogs, and cats

(continued on next page)

Table 4
(continued)

Clinical Condition	TCVM Pattern	Herbal Formula	Comments
Pruritus	External wind	External Wind[a]	Has been used in goats, sheep, llamas, alpacas, pigs, rabbits, small rodents, ferrets, and fish in addition to horses, dogs, and cats
Bleeding	Trauma, heat, or *Qi* deficiency	*Yunnan Bai Yao*	Has been used in goats, sheep, llamas, alpacas, pigs, rabbits, rodents, reptiles, giant pandas, and dolphins in addition to horses, dogs, and cats
Cystitis or urinary tract infection	Bladder damp heat	*Ba Zheng San* (Eight Righteous)	Has been used in goats, sheep, llamas, alpacas, pigs, rabbits, black bears, and giant pandas, in addition to horses, dogs, and cats
Kidney/urinary crystals or stones	Bladder damp heat	Crystal Stone Formula[a]	Has been used in rabbits, cows, and dolphins in addition to horses, dogs, and cats
Upper airway infections	Wind-heat	*Yin Qiao San*	Has been used in elephants, goats, sheep, llamas, alpacas, pigs, rabbits, birds, ferrets, reptiles, in addition to horses, dogs, and cats
Conjunctivitis, photophobia, pain in eyes	Liver fire flaring up	Haliotis formula[a] or *Ju Ming San*	Has been used in rabbits, cows and dolphins and other marine mammals in addition to horses and dogs
Chronic eye problems, keratoconjunctivitis sicca (KSC) or dry eye	Liver/kidney *Yin* deficiency	*Qi Ju Di Huang*	Has been used in rabbits, cows and dolphins in addition to horses and dogs
Aggression or irribibility along with GI disorders	Liver *Qi* stagnation	*Xiao Yao San*	Has been used in rabbits, small rodents, cows and dolphins in addition to horses and dogs
Hard or big cancer mass	Blood stasis	Stasis breaker[a]	Has been used in rabbits, small rodents, ferrets, reptiles, birds, cows, and dolphins in addition to horses, dogs, and cats
Small or soft tumor mass	Phlegm stagnation	Max's Formula[a]	Has been used in rabbits, birds, cows, and dolphins in addition to horses, dogs, and cats

[a] Manufactured and distributed by Jing-tang Herbal, Inc, Reddick, FL.

deficiency can also often be caused by undernutrition or poor diet quality. The common clinical signs of spleen *Qi* deficiency include diarrhea, loss of body weight, anorexia, lethargy, colic, nausea, or vomiting. Other common pediatric problems are poor development and growth, developmental orthopedic disease (DOD), and congenital diseases. Excessive pure breeding causes a limited gene pool, and consequently pure-bred animal breeds can be susceptible to a wide range of congenital

Table 5		
Most common *Tui-na* techniques used in exotic animals[16]		
Name	**Description of Technique**	**Actions and Indications**
Mo-fa Touching and rubbing	Touching or rubbing in a circular motion with the palm of the hand or one or more fingers	Improves blood and *Qi* circulation in subcutaneous tissues Pain in back, abdomen, limbs, and neck in rabbits, birds, and reptiles
Moo-fa Massaging/daubing	Up and down or side to side motion with the thumbs or fingers	Calms the spirit, benefits the eyes Anxiety, seizure, eye, and sinus problems in rabbits and birds
Rou-fa Rotary kneading	Rotary kneading using the heel of the palm on the superficial dermal tissues	Soothing and calming, reduces pain; Pain in neck, back, abdomen, and limbs in rabbits and birds
Ca-fa Rubbing	Rapid, linear, and mildly forceful rubbing firmly touching the skin using the palms of the hands for larger areas and the thumb for smaller areas	Heats the underlying tissue and is especially good for *Yang* deficiency Cold or damp *Bi* syndrome, diarrhea, renal failure and heart diseases due to *Yang/Qi* deficiency in rabbits and reptiles
An-fa Pressing	Applying gentle pressure to acupoints and *Ah-shi* points and other areas with the finger or palm (see *Dian-fa*)	Invigorates *Qi* and blood and relieves stagnation Pain in limbs and back in rabbits, birds, and reptiles
Dian-fa Knocking	Applying deeper pressure on acupoints and *Ah-Shi* points than *An-fa*, using the fingertips, knuckle, or elbow; also called acupressure or *shiatsu*	Invigorates blood, relieves pain, balances *Zang-fu* functions Pain in limbs and back in rabbits, birds, and reptiles
Dou-fa Shaking	Gently shake the limb, while holding it out stretched	Invigorates *Qi* and blood flow and relaxes the joints Pain in limbs in small mammals

diseases. In TCVM, poor development and growth, DOD, and congenital diseases are considered as kidney *Jing* deficiency.

In TCVM, infants and pediatrics are fragile with immature *Yin* and *Yang*. Their meridians and channels are not fully developed. Thus, needle-free acupuncture treatments including gentle *Tui-na* techniques are often used. The common and simple *Tui-na* techniques for exotic animals are listed in **Table 5**. Another needle-free method is to use low-level impulse laser therapy (LLLT) on the acupuncture points and meridians.[17]

Detailed information on the herbs for spleen *Qi* and kidney *Jing* deficiency is listed in **Table 6**. It is very challenging to give general guidelines of herbal dosage for all exotic pediatric as well as adult exotic animals. With more documented clinical experience and experimental studies of the TCVM treatment of exotic animals and pediatrics, the more accurate data will be found. Thus, this article represents an initial attempt to integrate TCVM in the exotic animal practice. The following information may help practitioners get some general idea of herbal dosage for exotic pediatrics.

Table 6
Herbs for exotic pediatrics

Pattern	Clinical Signs	Herbs
Spleen *Qi* deficiency	Diarrhea Loss of body weight Anorexia Colic Nausea or vomiting Pale tongue Deep and weak pulse	Four Gentlemen (*Si Jun Zi Tang*) is the primary herb Mume Powder (*Wu Mei San*) for diarrhea Eight Gentlemen for anorexia and weight loss Happy Earth for nausea or vomiting
Kidney *Jing* deficiency	Poor development and growth Developmental orthopedic disease (DOD) Congenital diseases Pale tongue Weak pulse	Epimedium powder is the primary one. *Yi Zhi Ren* for DOD

Mammal infants less than 14 days old are too young to use herbs, but herbs can be given to lactating mothers. The exotic animal baby can benefit from milk from the treated mother as commonly practiced in equines. For animals whose life span is 10 years or longer, herbs with lower dosage (about 1/10 normal dosage) can start to be orally given to infants of 15 to 30 days old. Herbs of one-fifth normal dosage can be orally given to infants age 31 to 60 days. Herbs of one-third normal dosages are given for age 61 to 120 days, one-half for age 121 to 180 days, and normal dosage for age 181 days or older.

For animals whose life span is less than 5 years, herbs with lower dosage (about one-eighth normal dosage) can start to be orally given to infants of 15 to 30 days old. Herbs of one-fourth normal dosage can orally be given for infants of 31 to 60 days, one-half normal dosages for 61 to 120 days, and full dosage to 121 days.

TCVM TREATMENT FOR SMALL MAMMAL PETS

Small mammal pets include rabbits, rats, mice, guinea pigs, ferrets, hamsters, and gerbils. The majority of health issues are caused by improper husbandry and diet. Geriatric small mammals are often presented with osteoarthritis, degenerative joint disease, or disk diseases. The TCVM treatment including acupuncture and herbs is very similar to that for the dog. Acupuncture points and herbal treatment can be extrapolated from canine transpositional points. Most small mammals can orally take herbal medications if mixed with a sweet liquid and offered or put via syringe into their mouths. Some of the herbivorous pets can be fed the herb itself, especially if the medicinal parts of the herb are the aerial portions of the plant.

The following case demonstrated how to use the TCVM treatment of small mammal pets like rabbits.

Case Study in Rabbits

Presentation
A 9-year-old 2.5-kg castrated male rabbit was presented with rear weakness for 2 years. He was diagnosed with lumbosacral disc disease 2 years ago.

Examination
He showed overall weakness and stayed in one spot most of the time. His haircoat around the hindquarters was urine soaked and foul-smelling because he could not move well. He was very stiff and weak in the rear limbs when forced to move. He was very sensitive around the lumbosacral junction on palpation. His tongue was pale purple, and his pulse was deep and weak.

Diagnosis
Bi syndrome due to kidney *Qi* deficiency.

Treatment
Acupuncture treatment

- Dry-needle: BL-23, BL-40
- Electroacupuncture (20 Hz for 10 minutes and 80–120 Hz for 10 minutes) at the following bilateral pairs of acupoints:
  ○ BL-11 + BL-20
  ○ BL-21 + BL-26
  ○ *Hua-tuo-jia-ji* at L-S
  ○ ST-36 + GB-34

Herbal medicine

- *Body Sore* (modified *Shen Tong Zhu Yu*), 0.2 g twice daily for 10 weeks, and then *Ba Ji San*, 0.2 g once daily for 6 months.

Outcome
The rabbit moved better and more frequently after 4-weekly acupuncture treatments and daily herbal medication of Body Sore. He was able to hop around after another 3 acupuncture treatments (1 session every 2 weeks) and 6 weeks of daily herbal medication. Acupuncture therapy was continued with 1 session every 1 to 3 months or as needed. He had had a great quality of life until 2 years later, when he was euthanized (**Fig. 1**).

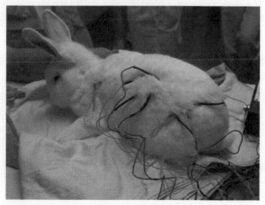

Fig. 1. Electroacupuncture in a rabbit. (*From* Xie H, Trevisanello L. Application of traditional Chinese veterinary medicine in exotic animals. Reddick (FL): Jing Tang Publishing; 2011; with permission.)

TCVM TREATMENT FOR BIRDS

Birds belong to *Yang* animals. Thus, a quiet (*Yin*) environment is an important factor to balance their health. Restraint of the avian patient should be the minimum necessary to protect the safety of both the bird and the handler/practitioner. Acupuncture procedure(s) should be as brief as possible as they are Yang and do not require too intense stimulation. Dry-needle and aquapuncture are the most commonly used techniques. Electroacupuncture stimulation is effective for the treatment of disc compression or nerve damage. Most herbal medicines have been used in domestic chickens and ducks safely and successfully in China and are used in many birds. Because of high body temperature, fast metabolism, and short gastrointestinal tract, herbal dosage for small birds (<2 kg) is often recommended at 0.5 to 1 g/kg body weight, which is higher than that for dogs and cats.

Case Study in Birds

Presentation
An 11-year-old 460-g male cockatoo was presented with rear limb weakness. He was rescued by the current owner who brought the bird to the local university wild animal service, which diagnosed the bird with a disc compression at C4-5 1 month earlier.

Examination
The bird had general weakness. He was very weak in the rear limbs (right side worse than left side). He was unable to fly and land. He could not eat by himself though his appetite was normal. His *Shen* was great.

Diagnosis
Wei syndrome due to *Qi* deficiency with local *Qi*-blood stagnation at the cervical region.

Treatment
Acupuncture treatment

- Dry needle: GV-20, *Bai-hui*, BL-11
- Electroacupuncture at the following pairs of acupoints (10 minutes of 20 Hz and 10 minutes of 80–120 Hz)
  - *Jing-jia-ji* at C4-5, bilateral (alternatively with GB-20 + GB-21)
  - *Jing-jia-ji* at C5-6, bilateral (alternatively with *Jing-jia-ji* at C3-4)
  - BL-23, bilateral
  - BL-26, bilateral
- He was treated with acupuncture one session per month for 3 months initially and then 1 session per 3 to 5 months.

Herbal medicine

- Cervical formula
  - 0.2 g was given orally, twice daily for 5 months.

Outcome and comment
The bird was able to fly about 1 m off the ground, land normally, and also eat by himself 1 year later after 8 acupuncture treatments and daily herbal medications. The bird had received acupuncture easily with the gentle hand over the neck for the first 3 sessions. Authors found that placing a stockinet over his head had worked very well to restrain this bird after he gained strength and started to avoid acupuncture (**Fig. 2**).

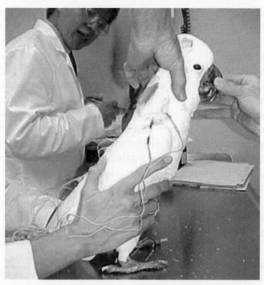

Fig. 2. Electro-acupuncture at in an 11-year-old cockatoo with a disc compression at C4-5. (*From* Xie H, Trevisanello L. Application of traditional Chinese veterinary medicine in exotic animals. Reddick (FL): Jing Tang Publishing; 2011; with permission.)

TCVM TREATMENT FOR REPTILES AND AMPHIBIANS

Reptiles are very *Yin* in nature compared to other animals. This diverse group of animals includes snakes, lizards, chelonians, and crocodilians, representing a staggering array of size, behavior, nutritional, and environmental requirements. It is critical to treatment success to research the husbandry requirements and natural history of the particular species being treated. The practitioner should also become familiar with restraint techniques appropriate for each species for their patients' as well as their own safety. Dry-needle acupuncture, aquapuncture, and electroacupuncture techniques can be used in most reptile patients. Care should be used to insert needles in between scales rather than penetrating them. In smaller, more active species, aquapuncture and laser acupuncture are most commonly used. Moxibustion can also be beneficial in the reptilian patient. The acupuncture points of lizards, crocodilians, and chelonians can be extrapolated from those of dogs and cats using transpositional acupuncture.[18,19] In snakes, acupuncture points are typically located by palpation, and the function of the points may be extrapolated based on their anatomic location and determining what organs or structures are present in the region of the point. Because of their elongated body structure, a single mammalian point may be represented by a region containing 4 or 5 points in snakes. Administration of herbs in these species will depend on the natural feeding habits of the patient. Small, active species and those that eat frequently can be given herbs once or twice daily, while larger species and those that eat infrequently should be dosed every other day. Some herbivorous species will readily consume powdered herbs offered as a top dressing on the food, and herbs in capsule or powder form can be hidden in the prey items of carnivores. Herbs can be suspended in compounding syrup for oral administration in any species, and this is often required in insectivores. Some reptiles will accept gentle *Tui-na* techniques. Food therapy is easily employed in herbivores but presents more of a challenge in carnivorous and insectivorous species. Gut loading prey items with the selected food items may help effect food therapy in these species.[19]

The amphibians represent another diverse and challenging group of exotics, including frogs and toads, salamanders and newts, and axolotls. They are relatively more *Yin* than mammalian and avian species but more *Yang* than most reptiles. Amphibian skin is extremely thin and delicate, and some amphibians possess venom glands, so practitioners should wear moistened powder-free gloves and use caution when handling these species. While some amphibians are very active, making acupuncture impractical, many can be treated using aquapuncture at anatomically located transpositional acupuncture points. *Tui-na* is impractical and not recommended for amphibians. Herbal formulas may be administered by compounding into a palatable slurry given by oral gavage or can be injected into prey items. Food therapy is accomplished by offering a greater variety of prey items or by gut loading of the items offered.[19]

Case Report in Reptiles

Presentation
A juvenile female iguana was found outdoors and presented for poor thrift, "shivering," and inability to move the pelvic limbs. The overall body color was dull and pale, and the iguana exhibited fine intention tremors when it attempted to move or when stressed during examination. It was unable to move the pelvic limbs and tail. The right pelvic limb appeared shorter than the left. The body condition was thin. Radiographically, multiple pathologic folding fractures were noted in the long bones and spinal vertebral bodies, and the overall bone density was considered poor. Clinicopathologic testing revealed hypocalcemia and elevated creatine phosphokinase (CPK) but no other significant abnormalities.

TCVM examination
The patient's *Shen* was fair, and the tongue was pale and slightly large with a sticky, clear coating. There was marked paresis and muscle atrophy of the pelvic limbs and delayed healing of old fractures.

Diagnosis
The iguana was diagnosed with kidney *Qi* deficiency based on the delayed fracture healing, pelvic limb paresis, pale wet tongue, and hindlimb paresis.

Treatment
The treatment principle was to tonify kidney *Qi*. A combination of electroacupuncture, dry-needle acupuncture, aquapuncture, and herbal therapy was used.

Acupuncture. Electroacupuncture was performed at 80 Hz, dense and disperse mode, for 20 minutes using the following pairs of points:

- LI-10 + ST-36 bilaterally
- BL-11 + BL-35 bilaterally

This was followed by aquapuncture with 0.05 mL of vitamin B12 at GB-39, SP-6, BL- 12, BL-23, and BL-25 bilaterally.

This treatment was repeated once weekly for 3 weeks.

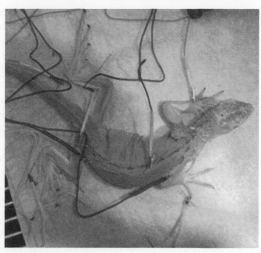

Fig. 3. Electroacupuncture in a green iguana.

Herbal medicine. Two herbal formulas, Chase Wind Penetrate Bone and Trauma 2 Formula (Golden Flower Chinese Herbs, Albuquerque, NM, USA), were prescribed and were given once daily for 30 days at a dose of 100 mg/kg.[20]

Outcome

The iguana's mobility and attitude improved significantly after the first acupuncture treatment, and after 1 month, the fractures had healed and tremors resolved. Minor abnormalities in pelvic limb gait persisted, but the lizard was otherwise normal.

Comments

Excellent husbandry practices were also critical to the outcome of this case. The iguana in this case was housed in an aquarium with a 90°F basking area, with the cool side of the aquarium at 80°F to allow for self-regulation of temperature. A full-spectrum ultraviolet A/B mercury vapor light was suspended over the cage approximate 18 inches above the basking area and left on 24 hours per day for 1 month. Dietary recommendations included feeding a mixed salad of fresh, preferably organic produce daily, including parsley, turnip greens, watercress, kale and collards, carrots, apples, and sweet potatoes. Supplementation with oral calcium gluconate was continued throughout the treatment period (**Fig. 3**).

TCVM TREATMENT FOR MARINE MAMMALS, ORNAMENTAL FISH, SEA LIONS, AND SEALS

Treating animals that reside in an aquatic environment provides a new and interesting challenge for the practitioner. As with most exotics, the species differences in habitat, dietary and foraging preferences, anatomy, and species compatability in community displays can be overwhelming. Assessment of water quality, movement, and aeration must also be taken into account. The practitioner must also be familiar with safe methods of capture and restraint for each species. For most commonly encountered ornamental fishes, dry-needle acupuncture, and aquapuncture techniques can be safely accomplished. Acupuncture point-like areas have been identified in the skin of zebrafish, and a schematic representation of these points has been published.[21] Acupuncture needles should be inserted in between scales. As fish have inelastic skin, when aquapuncture is used, light digital pressure should be briefly applied to the site to prevent the injected solution from seeping out through the hole produced by the hypodermic needle. Insertion of needles along the lateral line of fishes should be avoided. Sedation may be needed to safely restrain fish for acupuncture. Herbal medications may be administered by incorporation into a medicated gel diet[22,23] as has been previously described. This same diet may also be used to incorporate foods selected for food therapy or selected items may be offered normally. *Tui-na* is impractical in fish and is not recommended.

Information regarding the use of TCVM in marine mammals is limited. Point location has been described in Atlantic bottle-nosed dolphins.[24,25] LLLT has been used to stimulate acupuncture points around the eye as an adjunct therapy in treating ophthalmic disease in sea lions.[26] A thorough knowledge of the anatomy and natural history of the species being treated is absolutely essential before undertaking any course of therapy. While often well-trained, many aquatic mammals cannot be easily treated without sedation. Safety of the patient, handlers, and practitioner must be the primary concern and may limit the treatment options. While herbal therapy and food therapy are applicable to these species, many are kept in collections with strictly controlled diets and treatment regimens that may not allow for the use of these treatment modalities. Excellent communication with keepers and handlers is crucial for treatment success.

Case Report in Fish

Presentation

A mature koi presented for traumatic wounds around the mouth and head, and severe bruising along the epaxial area after being attacked and pulled out of the pond by an unidentified predator. The fish was lethargic, sinking in the water column, and had limited mobility with a slight bend into a "C" shape toward the left. The koi normally responded to the presence of its owner by surfacing to accept food treats but would not respond to the owner at the time of presentation. The fish was placed in a hospital tank and treated conventionally with antibiotics and anti-inflammatory medication for 1 week with only minor improvement.

TCVM examination

The koi was lethargic with marked bruising in the epaxial area and traumatic wounds to the face and head. Its *Shen* was poor and it was lethargic and inappetant.

Diagnosis

The koi was diagnosed with *Qi* and blood stasis based on the bruising and trauma. A diagnosis of spleen *Qi* deficiency was also made based on the lethargy and lack of appetite.

Treatment

Acupuncture. Dry-needle acupuncture was performed with needles inserted to a depth of 2 mm with an even technique and retained for 15 minutes. Points were chosen based on palpation of sensitive areas along the edge of the epaxial musculature, consistent with the BL meridian of other species. This treatment was repeated once daily for 3 days.

Conventional treatment with antibiotics and anti-inflammatory medication was continued throughout this time period.

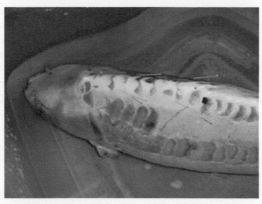

Fig. 4. Dry-needle acupuncture in a koi.

Herbal medicine. Aloe vera (*Lu hui*) was applied topically to the wounds on the head and face, directly from the leaves of the aloe plant. This was repeated 3 times daily for 7 days.

Outcome

After 2 weeks of hospitalization and treatment, the koi was more mobile and began to approach the surface of the water to accept food from the owner. It was discharged to the owners' care and was housed in a hospital tank for an additional week of observation before being returned to the pond.

Comments

Caring for aquatics in outdoor displays requires special attention to predator exclusion. Netting draped over the pond surface may help exclude raptors and other avian predators, while fencing or other measures may be needed to protect against predation by mammals. Other hazards to consider include the risk of lightning strike or electric shock from malfunctioning pumps or filters (**Fig. 4**).

SUMMARY

Exotic animals, both pediatric and adult, are amenable to TCVM diagnosis and respond well to the TCVM treatment including acupuncture and herbal medicine. With more documented clinical experience and experimental studies of the TCVM treatment of exotic animals, more diseases in more species will be identified to be effectively treated with the TCVM.

REFERENCES

1. Yu C. Traditional Chinese veterinary medicine. 2nd edition. Beijing (China): China Agriculture Press; 1985. p. 1–6.
2. Xie H, Chrisman C. Equine acupuncture: from ancient art to modern validation. Am J Trad Chin Vet Med 2009;4(2):1–4.
3. Xie H, Preast V. Traditional Chinese veterinary medicine: fundamental principles. Reddick (FL): Jing Tang; 2002. p. 1–25.
4. McCluggage D. Acupuncture for the avian patients. In Schoen A, editor. Veterinary acupuncture. 2nd edition. St Louis (MO): Mosby; 2001. p. 307–32.

5. Zhao CJ, Fan YS, Lu LP, et al. Effects of moxibustion at "Shenque" (CV 8) on superoxide dismutase (SOD) in rabbits with kidney-yang deficiency. Zhongguo Zhen Jiu 2011;31(4):342–6 [in Chinese].

6. Xie H. How to use acupuncture for elephants. Proceedings of the North American Veterinary Conference: Small Animal Edition, volume 17. Orlando (FL), January 17–21, 2004. p. 1457–8.

7. Cantwell SL, Brooks DE, Xie H, et al. Electro-acupuncture to decrease intraocular pressure in Rhesus monkeys with chronic glaucoma. Proceedings of the annual meeting of the Association for Research in Vision and Ophthalmology (ARVO). Fort Lauderdale (FL): Investigative Ophthalmology & Visual Science; 2007. p. 48.

8. Wang LT. Integrative therapies for the treatment of constipation in the Giant Panda. J Trad Chin Vet Med 2007;3:63–4.

9. McCaskill L. "Tora the Tiger" and TCVM. TCVM News 2011;Spring(14):8–9.

10. Haddad MA. *Tui-na* as an adjunct treatment for pain control and rehabilitation in a jaguar with suspected nutritional secondary hyperparathyroidism. Am J Trad Chin Vet Med 2009;4:47–51.

11. Scognamillo-Szabó MV, Santos AL, Olegário MM, et al. Acupuncture for locomotor disabilities in a South American red-footed tortoise (Geochelone carbonaria): a case report. Acupunct Med 2008;26(4):243–7.

12. Niu L, Wedemeyer L, Hightman S. Application of traditional Chinese veterinary medicine in other exotic species. In: Xie H, Wedemeyer L, editors. Practical traditional Chinese veterinary medicine. Reddick (FL): Jing Tang Publishing; 2012, in press.

13. Yu C. Chinese veterinary acupuncture and moxibustion [in Chinese]. Beijing (China): China Agricultural Press; 1995. p. 1–6.

14. Wang K, Liu HF, Zhou WH. [Effects of catgut embedding at "Zusanli" (ST 36) and "Shenshu" (BL 23) on morphine analgesic tolerance and locomotor sensitization in the rat]. Zhongguo Zhen Jiu 2008;28(7):509–13 [in Chinese].

15. Yang YQ, Huang GY. [Study on effects of acupuncture on mice dysmenorrhea model and the mechanism]. Zhongguo Zhen Jiu 2008;28(2):119–21 [in Chinese].

16. Xie H, Ferguson B, Deng X. Application of Tui-na in veterinary medicine. 2nd edition. Reddick (FL): Chi Institute; 2007. p. 1–94, 129–32.

17. Petermann U. Comparison of pre- and post-treatment pain scores of twenty-one horses with laminitis treated with acupoint and topical low level laser therapy. Am J Trad Chin Vet Med 2011;6(1):13–5.

18. Ferguson B. Alternative and complementary veterinary therapies. In: Mader D, editor. Reptile medicine and surgery. 2nd edition. St. Louis (MO): Elsevier; 2006. p. 426–41.

19. Eckermann-Ross C. Reptiles and amphibians. In: Xie H, Trevisanello L, editors. Application of traditional Chinese veterinary medicine in exotic animals. Reddick (FL): Jing Tang Publishing; 2011. p. 159–208.

20. Scott J, Monda L, Heuertz J. Clinical guide to commonly used Chinese herbal formulas. 5th ed. Placitas (NM): Herbal Medicine Press; 2011. p. 10, 107.

21. Jin ZG, Jing XH, Li JW, et al. Preliminary observation of acupoint-like and meridian-like structures on the body surface of the zebrafish [in Chinese]. Zhongguo Zhen Jiu 2007;27(2):117–9.

22. Grazek JB. Aquariology–master volume: the science of fish health management. Morris Plains (NJ): Tetra Press; 1992. p. 218–74.

23. Eckermann-Ross C. Ornamental fishes. In: Xie H, Trevisanello L, editors. Application of traditional Chinese veterinary medicine in exotic animals. Reddick (FL): Jing Tang Publishing; 2011. p. 237–49.

24. Clemmons-Chevis C. Preliminary study: transposition of meridians and acupoints from canine and equine to the Atlantic bottlenose dolphin. Proceeding of the Twenty-Fifth Annual International Congress on Veterinary Acupuncture. San Antonio (TX): International Society of Veterinary Acupuncture; 2009. p. 111–27.
25. Clemmons-Chevis C. A preliminary study on the transposistion of meridians and acupuncture points from the canin and equine species to the Atlantic bottlenose dolphin, Tursiops truncatus. Am J Trad Chin Vet Med 2007;2:23–32.
26. Eckermann-Ross C. Pinnipeds (sea lions and seals). In: Xie H, Trevisanello L, editors. Application of traditional Chinese veterinary medicine in exotic animals. Reddick (FL): Jing Tang Publishing; 2011. p. 231–6.

Index

Note: Page numbers of article titles are in **boldface** type.

V

W

Moving?

Make sure your subscription moves with you!

To notify us of your new address, find your **Clinics Account Number** (located on your mailing label above your name), and contact customer service at:

Email: journalscustomerservice-usa@elsevier.com

800-654-2452 (subscribers in the U.S. & Canada)
314-447-8871 (subscribers outside of the U.S. & Canada)

Fax number: 314-447-8029

Elsevier Health Sciences Division
Subscription Customer Service
3251 Riverport Lane
Maryland Heights, MO 63043

*To ensure uninterrupted delivery of your subscription, please notify us at least 4 weeks in advance of move.

Printed and bound by CPI Group (UK) Ltd, Croydon, CR0 4YY

03/10/2024

01040458-0003